Eating Your Way to Better Health

The Prostate Forum Nutrition Guide

Charles E. Myers, Jr., MD
Sara Sgarlat Steck, RT
Rose Sgarlat Myers, PT, PhD

Rivanna Health Publications, Inc.
Charlottesville

Second Printing 2000

ISBN 0-9676129-0-X

LCCN

foreword

October in Charlottesville indulges all one's senses and appetites; the trees are gloriously colored, the scent of the air is at once crisp and spiced, leaves crunch underfoot, and the wind gusts seem to come out of nowhere. And, of course, the tastes of the fall harvest are to me unequaled. It was over hors d'oeuvres in a beautiful Virginia country inn last October that Bill and I engaged in an animated discussion about food with Rose, Snuffy, and their neighbors. While we certainly didn't exhaust the subject, we did cover such topics as the proper growing conditions for different varieties of exotic mushrooms, vegetable gardens, favorite preparations of beets, the purveyors we use at our restaurant for seafood and produce, favorite grains, and so forth. We came away from that evening impressed with Snuffy and Rose's knowledge of, and enthusiasm for, fine food. We were convinced that the cookbook they were writing would be a great resource.

It is another amazing October day that, wearing many hats, I sit down to write a few words about *Eating Your Way to Better Health - The Prostate Forum Nutrition Guide.* As a writer, I am filled with admiration for the time and effort that the authors have invested in this project. I am honored to be a small part. As a restaurateur, I have a great appreciation for the authors' creative approaches to wonderful food, and their mindfulness of the full range of senses to which such food must appeal. As a patient, I am grateful to know that there are physicians in leadership positions, who value patient empowerment. As a breast cancer survivor, I have experienced my own personal quest for an answer to this disease. And as a volunteer and advocate for the University of Virginia Cancer Center, I have become familiar with the work of so many brilliant researchers, who are approaching cancer from every conceivable angle in a determined effort to quash its power. By articulating so clearly the impact of diet and nutrition on the body's defenses, and the science behind different food choices, by creating appetizing recipes and providing thorough instructions, Snuffy, Sara, and Rose offer prostate cancer patients an agreeable way in which they can join forces with their health care providers and participate in their own well being.

When Bill and I developed the concept for our restaurant, Hamiltons' at First & Main, we described our menu as "contemporary American cuisine." By contemporary, we meant innovative preparations of the finest available foods in keeping with current nutritional trends. For us,

"American" implied incorporating the foods and flavors of the many cultures that make up the "Melting Pot." Cuisine meant to us that our dishes would be prepared with the greatest integrity and presented with attention not only to flavors, but also to textures and design. Our menu is relatively short and changes frequently in its entirety. While Hamiltons' is not primarily a vegetarian restaurant, the menu always includes several vegetarian, often Vegan, appetizers and entrees. Of particular interest to us is the fact that the sales of our culturally themed Vegetarian Plate have nearly always surpassed any other item on the menu. In our research for this dish, we remain fascinated by the variety of traditional combinations of vegetable proteins that existed in the cuisine's of other cultures long before we recognized their nutritional value. *Eating Your Way to Better Health - The Prostate Forum Nutrition Guide* is an excellent reference for those who wish to introduce these healthful dishes into their own homes.

Kate and Bill Hamilton
Hamiltons' at First & Main
Director, Advisory Board, University of Virginia Cancer Center
Charlottesville, VA
October, 1999

Dedication:

For our subscribers
who inspired us
to write this book.

Acknowledgements

The authors offer their special thanks and gratitude to Jewell W. Loring and Keith W. Loring for their many hours of copy editing. We are deeply indebted to them for correcting our grammar and punctuation. Our thanks to Stephen J. Druhe and Sara Sgarlat Steck, for the picture on our cover and to Louise Spangler, Carl Spangler, and Maryann Brown for cover design.

We also thank John C. Wayland for his support in our office while this work was on-going.

Thanks to Kemper Conwell for her assistance in formatting this book.

Preface

The idea for this book germinated after the first six issues of the **PROSTATE FORUM** were published. For many years Dr. Myers' has advocated a prudent low-fat diet for his prostate cancer patients. His diet guidelines are based on recent scientific literature.

Rose Sgarlat Myers, PT, PhD, and Sara Sgarlat Steck, RT, have translated Dr. Myers' ideas into good-tasting recipes for a healthy lifestyle. The recipes are easy to prepare and adequate background is given to assist even the new cook. We think some of the recipes in this book will become your favorites.

The authors have followed the intent of these guidelines in their own lives for many years. The process from meat-eater to vegetarian has been gradual. We did not give up all meat overnight. In fact, we sometimes still enjoy a good salmon fillet or baked chicken. The guidelines are meant to help you change your eating habits to sustain your life.

Eating Your Way to Better Health—The Prostate Forum Nutrition Guide is not intended to serve as a guide to weight-loss, but a guide to a healthy lifestyle in which food is still good and tasty.

Rose Sgarlat Myers, PT, PhD
Sara Sgarlat Steck, RT
Charles E. Myers, Jr., MD

Eating Your Way to Better Health

The Prostate Forum
Nutrition Guide

Recipes for a Healthy Life: So You Thought It Was Hard?!

Chapter9:

Chapter 10:

Chapter 11:

Chapter 12:

Chapter 13:
    Side Dishes
    Breakfast Dishes

Chapter 14:

Appendix

Chapter 1:
Taking Ownership of Your Disease

There is a natural tendency for patients to accept the advice of the medical profession. The idea is that you have put yourself in the hands of a highly competent professional whom you trust to make appropriate decisions about your treatments. This is not always a good idea. There are many options available in the treatment of prostate cancer and no one physician is an expert in the full range of possibilities. Also, there is a real tendency for physicians to favor the approach they use – they are proud of their skills.

You are a unique patient with personal preferences and goals. *Two medically equivalent treatments may not be equally beneficial for you.* In fact, some patients may prefer a treatment that is less likely to cure them because they find the side effects of a more aggressive treatment unacceptable. Others are willing to risk any side effect from an untested new treatment for the possibility of cure. Only you can make these decisions, not your physician, and only you should develop an integrated program to fight this disease and maintain optimal health.

A good place to begin is to rethink the meaning of health and disease. In medicine, we have long known that health is not just the absence of disease. In truth, most adults who seem healthy have several disease processes ongoing. The young athlete in his twenties you see winning a race may already have early stage atherosclerosis. In fact, he may also have early prostate cancer! These diseases do not prevent him from being an example of vigorous health. This picture of health may continue for many years or even decades before the silent disease processes become apparent. The key point is that happy, healthy, productive people achieve this state despite the presence of disease. You can be the same way. Just because you have been diagnosed with prostate cancer does not mean that you can not feel healthy, enjoy your life, and radiate good health. The first step is to take ownership of your disease and its management. Then you must craft a program that emphasizes health and minimizes disability.

1

These are the steps for you to take ownership of your disease. Develop an understanding of prostate cancer and the various paths this disease can take. In collaboration with your physicians, use this information to craft a treatment plan that fits your medical situation and your personal goals. Once this is in place, make certain changes in your life that only you can accomplish. One critical factor is to become physically active. Set up a regular program of exercise designed to promote good balance, strength, and endurance so that you can enjoy life.

You also need to attend to your emotional needs. Here, family and friends play a major role, because prostate cancer effects the entire family. We find that patient support-groups, such as Man-to-Man or US TOO!, make a major contribution to patient happiness. There is something special about the interaction among men and women who share the diagnosis of prostate cancer.

Finally, alter your diet to help you control prostate cancer. The goal of this book is to explain what we know about diet and prostate cancer and what you can do about it.

What can you expect if you adopt the dietary recom-mendations listed in this book? Many patients report to us that they experience an increase in their energy level and feel better than they have in years. You will be able to withstand the various treatments used to treat prostate cancer much better. For example, hormonal therapy commonly causes men to gain five to fifteen pounds. A program of exercise and the low-fat diet we recommend will counter that trend. We have seen men lose, rather than gain, five to ten pounds while on hormonal therapy because they have altered their diet and developed an exercise program.

The benefits of the dietary program outlined in this book have been shown to reduce the risk of other diseases in addition to prostate cancer. Published clinical trials have documented that the dietary patterns we recommend will also reduce your risk of dying of heart disease and other cancers. Many patients tell us they feel healthier now than before they were diagnosed with prostate cancer. Families who adopt our recommendations will lead healthier lives.

Chapter 2:
Evidence-Based Nutrition and Prostate Cancer

A few years ago, prostate cancer was a disease that men did not talk about and it received little attention from the scientific community. Physicians treated this cancer with little hope of success and usually communicated negative feelings to their patients.

A dramatic change is occurring. Prostate cancer patient support groups are doing a great deal to educate patients about treatment options. The federal government and the CaP CURE Foundation have dramatically increased funding for research on all aspects of prostate cancer. As a result, hardly a week goes by without a major news story on prostate cancer. The Internet provides patients access to a wide range of information and resources about prostate cancer.

One result is that patients and their families may be overwhelmed with information about prostate cancer. Anyone can claim to be an expert on prostate cancer and set up an Internet web site. Much of the information and advice available on the Internet is wrong and even may be dangerous. This is especially true of advice on the role of nutrition in the prevention and management of prostate cancer.

In contrast to the dubious information being promoted at some Internet sites, there is a growing body of sound science and clinical investigation that documents a link between diet and the natural history of prostate cancer. Most of this information is contained in papers written by scientists for other scientists in a language with a rather remote relationship to everyday English. Some of the more dramatic results have been mentioned in the media, but a large number of interesting studies remain unnoticed.

In our newsletter, **PROSTATE FORUM**, we try to keep our readers informed about all advances in prostate cancer treatment. The most popular topic we cover is diet and nutrition. Our subscribers have repeatedly asked us to write a cookbook to help them develop and prepare a healthy diet.

The goals of this book are:

- to review what we know about the role diet plays in the biology of prostate cancer

- to provide a list of nutritional supplements that may be of help to you

- to warn you about certain dietary practices and nutritional supplements that may <u>fuel</u> the growth of prostate cancer or harm your health in other ways

- to provide instructions and recipes that will help you use nutritional information, intelligently on a daily basis

Evidence-Based Nutrition

It is important for you to understand how we evaluate the scientific literature on the link between diet and prostate cancer. We are looking for dietary items that document a positive impact of diet on the incidence of prostate cancer or the number of deaths attributed to prostate cancer. The most convincing type of evidence is a clinical trial in which a group of patients are randomly allocated to receive or not receive a component of the diet. These trials typically contain more than 1,000 subjects. These trials must run for a long enough period of time to gauge the impact of diet. This can take five to ten years. We find it more convincing if design of the trial and its results are also supported by sound laboratory science on the factors governing the growth and spread of prostate cancer. Finally, it is best that any positive trial be run a second time to confirm the result, although this process can easily take ten to twenty years and take millions of dollars to execute.

Large randomized trials are usually preceded by what are called Phase I and II clinical trials. In a Phase I clinical trial, the dose of the drug or nutrient is given in a series of increasing amounts to determine the safest and most effective dose to use for subsequent work. This is followed by a Phase II clinical trial, in which a group of patients are treated identically and the impact of treatment determined. This study design is quite common throughout medicine. In fact, a majority of the papers published on the treatment of prostate cancer with surgery, radiation therapy, or chemotherapy fit this design. In prostate cancer favorable results with the standard treatment approaches usually have not led to the design and conduct of large randomized controlled trials. This is in contrast to nutritional research in which we have several large randomized controlled trials that document the impact of nutrition on prostate cancer. Evidence supporting the role of nutrition in the treatment of prostate cancer is now stronger than that supporting the use of these other approaches.

There are several lines of evidence that are valuable even though they fall somewhat short of this ideal. One common design is to look at a large population and determine which dietary items are more or less common in men who develop prostate cancer. Studies using this design suggest that the risk of prostate cancer may be altered by reducing consumption of fat or increasing consumption of a range of items such as green tea, soybeans, and tomato products. The best studies of this type ask the patient to identify on an ongoing basis what they are eating and may even involve measuring the levels of a nutrient in the blood or urine. Unfortunately, many studies ask the study participant to remember past dietary patterns. How accurately can you remember your consumption of various dietary fats a week over the past five years?

As we discuss each dietary item, we will mention the evidence that supports its use. In many cases, the evidence is far from complete. Some advocates of evidence-based medicine argue that you should not take any drug if its value has not been proven. We think this strict approach makes little sense when applied to many issues in nutrition. We think a sounder approach is to weigh the potential benefits and risks before making a decision. In several cases we will discuss, the potential benefits are large and the risks nonexistent. The consumption of cooked tomatoes provides a good example. The proof of their value in prevention or management of prostate cancer is quite incomplete. Would you stop eating cooked tomato products just because we lack final proof of their value in the management of prostate cancer? What is the risk to you if you eat cooked tomatoes and subsequent randomized controlled trials show that they really do not prevent prostate cancer? You will still have had the chance to enjoy a good plate of spaghetti!

The rules we used in designing our recommendations for this book are:

Rule #1: <u>All cancers are not alike.</u> Leukemias, lymphomas, and cancers of the breast, lung, colon, and prostate are all different diseases. Nutritional practices that may be wise for patients with other cancers do not necessarily benefit prostate cancer patients. For example, flaxseed oil may lessen the risk of heart disease and may be of value to people with colon or breast cancer, but the scientific evidence we have available today suggests that this oil may dramatically increase the risk of metastatic prostate cancer. Issues like this have led us to look for specific information on the link between nutrition and the risk of prostate cancer.

Rule #2: <u>The recommendations we make are basically good for your general health as well as your prostate gland.</u> We have carefully reviewed all of our recommendations for their impact on general health as well as on common diseases such as heart disease, high blood pressure, and diabetes. There are components that may help prostate cancer, but increase the risk of other diseases. Where this is the case, we will warn you.

Rule #3: <u>Dietary recommendations must be attractive, tasty, and easy to prepare.</u> Some of the foods thought to lower the risk of prostate cancer include cooked tomatoes, grains, and beans — especially soybeans. Diets that incorporate these elements include those of the Mediterranean and the Orient. Judging from the popularity of Italian, Greek, Japanese, and Chinese restaurants, most Americans find these cuisines appealing. The recipes in this book are drawn from the culinary traditions of those cultures.

Rule #4: <u>Judgment is required when the information is incomplete or contradictory.</u> All too often, clinical studies on diet and cancer lead to contradictory results. This is particularly the case with dietary fat and prostate cancer. We have several ways to approach this problem. The first is to recognize that not all clinical studies are of equal quality. We have yet to see a clinical study without some fault. This is so because clinical research is very complex. Some studies have fewer defects or the defects may be relatively unimportant. Second, we are more confident if the results of the clinical trial are consistent with sound laboratory research. We are most confident when quality clinical trials and laboratory studies provide a consistent view of how this cancer behaves. A good example of this is the role of antioxidants in prostate cancer prevention and treatment.

Chapter 3:
Prostate Cancer—A Unique Disease

To understand the role of nutrition in prostate cancer management you first need to understand prostate cancer. Prostate cancer passes through a series of stages on its way to becoming a lethal disease. At the beginning, it grows, often slowly, within the confines of the prostate gland. During this time the disease can be cured with surgery or radiation therapy. At some point, the cancer cells develop the capacity to leave the prostate gland and migrate to the bone and other organs. Once the cancer has begun growing in the bone, it is difficult or impossible to cure. For this reason, it is important to do everything possible to prevent the cancer from spreading out of the prostate gland into the bone.

Prostate cancer is the most common cancer in humans. Autopsy studies have been done on men who died from other causes. Between birth and age 10, prostate cancer is essentially absent. However, between ages 10 and 20, a small percent of men will develop prostate cancer. By ages 50 to 60, approximately half the men will have cancer present in their gland. Over ages 70 to 80, between 80 and 100% will have prostate cancer. These numbers indicate that between 20 and 30 million American males have prostate cancer. In the United States, this pattern appears regardless of race or ethnic origin. The same pattern is seen in Japan and most other countries that have been studied. In all of these studies, there is no evidence that race, ethnic origin, geography or diet alter the risk of developing prostate cancer.

While 20 to 30 million men in America may have cancer in their prostate glands, only 40-50,000 will die of prostate cancer each year. The simple fact is that most of the cancers detected at autopsy were small and were growing so slowly that men died from other causes before the cancer caused any problems. It is apparent that this is one cancer that has difficulty developing the tools needed to grow fast and spread throughout the body. If we can make it even more difficult for the cancer to develop these tools, we may be able to reduce the death rate from this disease. There is evidence that diet may be able to do just that.

Autopsy studies indicate that prostate cancer is just as common in Japan as it is in the United States, but death rates from prostate cancer are 90% lower in Japan. This appears to be true throughout the Orient. In the United States prostate cancer is just as common in Caucasians and African-Americans, however, death rates are much lower among Caucasians. When Japanese men move to the United States, their death rate from prostate cancer begins to increase toward the number observed among Caucasians. These observations suggest that elements in the environment play a role in the development of rapidly growing prostate cancer which is able to spread throughout the body.

These findings triggered intense interest in the scientific community and resulted in a flood of new information about the relationship between diet and the development of life-threatening prostate cancer. The emerging consensus is that nutrition has little influence on whether men develop prostate cancer that grows slowly and does not spread beyond the prostate gland. The evidence we have *suggests that nutrition has a major impact on whether the cancer develops the capacity to grow rapidly and spread throughout the body.*

You should not expect a prostate cancer healthy diet to prevent you from getting prostate cancer: that will happen to nearly every man if he lives long enough. What you can expect is that a prostate healthy diet may lower your risk of dying of this disease. Even if you have wide spread prostate cancer, a prostate healthy diet may help you to live longer.

It is important not to have unrealistic expectations about the impact of diet on your risk of developing or dying of prostate cancer. The most impressive clinical trial on diet to date tested the impact of the mineral, selenium. Men who took selenium experienced greater than a 60% decline in prostate cancer deaths. While this is impressive, it is far short of a 100% decline. The point is that regardless of how healthy your live-style, you can still get prostate cancer and die from it. While our understanding of this relationship is still incomplete, what we know today is sufficient to reduce the risk of dying of prostate cancer by more than 50%.

It is critical that you and your doctor develop a program to detect prostate cancer early. Screening should begin at least by age 40 if you have a family history of prostate cancer. Otherwise, you should begin screening by age 50.

DIETARY COMPONENTS THAT ALTER THE DEVELOPMENT OF PROSTATE CANCER

We will now discuss specific chemicals in the diet that appear to have activity against human prostate cancer.

Dietary Fats

There have been dramatic scientific advances in our understanding of how dietary fat promotes the <u>development</u> of prostate cancer. We now know that components of dietary fat also stimulate the <u>spread</u> and <u>growth</u> of human prostate cancer.

As cancers grow, they need to form new blood vessels to supply added food and oxygen. A component of fat can dramatically enhance new blood vessel formation by prostate cancer cells. The immune response to cancer involves both natural killer cells and T cells that are also able to kill cancer cells. Prostate cancer cells can use dietary fat to produce chemicals capable of killing or disabling both of these immune cells. In summary, certain dietary fats allow the cancer cells to grow and survive, evade the immune system, and spread to distant parts of the body.

What Is Fat?

Fat is made up of two parts: glycerin and fatty acids. Glycerin has three attachment points for fatty acids and acts as a backbone for the synthesis of fat. The fatty acids are responsible for the properties of different fats. For example, olive oil is rich in oleic acid, while cocoa butter is rich in stearic and palmitic acids. When we talk about an individual fat being good or bad for your health, we are really talking about the effects of the different fatty acids in that fat.

10

There are a large number of individual fatty acids and it is worth understanding how these fatty acids differ. Fatty acids are composed of a carbon chain that ends in an acid group. The fatty acids important for this discussion consist of straight chains containing between 10 and 22 carbons lined up in a row.

Saturated and Unsaturated Fat

A saturated fatty acid is made up of a straight chain of carbon atoms with a single link between each carbon in the chain. Monounsaturated fatty acids have a double link between two of the carbons. A polyunsaturated fatty acid has more than one double link.

Patients with heart disease are often advised to increase their intake of polyunsaturated fats because it will decrease their cholesterol. As you will see, this recommendation may increase your risk of developing metastatic prostate cancer.

Omega-6 and Omega-3

Many authorities have told us that "omega-6" fatty acids are dangerous for us, while "omega-3" fatty acids can improve your health. What are omega-3 and omega-6 fatty acids? We just mentioned that polyunsaturated fats have a double link between two carbons. The omega number *simply describes where along the carbon chain you will find the first double link:* it is three, six or nine carbons from the end of the fatty acid.

The most important thing for you to remember is that omega-6 fatty acids can be converted into very powerful hormones that play major roles in human disease. The hormones derived from omega-6 fatty acids foster the development of high blood pressure, psoriasis, stroke, heart attacks, asthma, rheumatoid arthritis, and colon cancer. These fatty acids are also important in the genesis of a wide range of other cancers.

Corn oil is an example of dietary fat rich in omega-6 fatty acids, while fish and flaxseed oil are rich in omega-3 fatty acids. We will now discuss how one omega-6 fatty acid, arachidonic acid, fosters the progression of human prostate cancer. We will also tell you how to reduce the amount of arachidonic acid in your diet.

Essential Fatty Acid Deficiency

If you go to a health food store, you will see capsules that are claimed to supply "essential fatty acids." Certain polyunsaturated fats are needed for the normal function of your body: examples are arachidonic, linoleic, and linolenic acid. If humans or most other mammals eat a diet free of these fatty acids, they will become sick and even die. Fortunately, except for premature infants and people lacking important parts of their gut because of disease or surgery, humans cannot become essential-fatty-acid deficient on a normal diet.

As with many important nutrients, such as vitamins A and D, you can get sick if you take too large a dose of essential fatty acids. Most Americans suffer from the side effects of too much of each essential fatty acid. In the previous section, we listed some of the diseases linked to omega-6 fatty acids. In each case, excess intake of essential omega-6 fatty acids increases the risk of disease or increases the severity of the disease. We think the evidence strongly suggests that one of these side effects might be metastatic prostate cancer. The most important message is that you should only take essential fatty acid supplements if your physician thinks you have one of the uncommon medical conditions likely to cause a deficiency in these fatty acids.

Fat and Prostate Cancer

There are enormous controversies about the link between diet and the risk of metastatic prostate cancer. The situation is so contentious that you can almost pick studies to support any conclusion you might favor. There are a number of reasons for this situation. Most studies use crude methods such as requiring people to remember what they ate in the past or measuring the disappearance of certain foodstuffs from the economy of various countries. The determination of prostate cancer incidence is also quite rough because different cultures vary in their willingness to report prostate cancer accurately as a cause of death. Given these problems, only the strongest associations between diet and prostate cancer will be reliable. One of these is the association between a diet rich in animal products, especially red meat, and prostate cancer, suggesting a strong link between a component of meat and the risk of prostate cancer.

Of course, not all studies of prostate cancer and diet are of equal quality. The best type of study would be a clinical trial in which patients were randomly assigned to diets high or low in specific fats. Trials that fit this description are currently in progress. Until they are done, we have to use our next best option. In our opinion, some of the best studies on diet and prostate cancer are those published by the investigators at the Harvard School of Public Health. These investigators conducted two trials: one involving physicians and a second involving other health care professionals. In both studies, information on diet was conducted prospectively and did not depend on people accurately recalling the composition of their diet in the distant past. The information from the two studies indicates that dietary fat did not influence the risk of <u>localized</u> prostate cancer, but did increase the risk of <u>metastatic</u> prostate cancer. When they examined specific foods, red meat, dairy fat, egg yolks, and creamy salad dressings emerged as significant risk factors for metastatic disease.

Animal Fat

One fatty acid, <u>arachidonic</u> acid, is present in much greater concentration in animal products. Vegans are people who eat no animal products and they typically have arachidonic acid levels that are 10-30% of those found in meat-eaters. This fatty acid is known to have a dramatic impact on the behavior of cancer cells, including cancer of the prostate (Figure 1). Arachidonic acid has been shown to enhance prostate cancer growth, stimulate its spread, and to facilitate its ability to form new blood vessels. Arachidonic acid products have also been shown to kill cells of the immune system involved in the control of cancer.

While a diet rich in meat can supply large amounts of arachidonic acid, most mammals can also produce their own. The "essential" fatty acid, linoleic acid, can be converted to arachidonic acid. Linoleic acid is commonly present in large amounts in most plant oils. In most animals used in diet

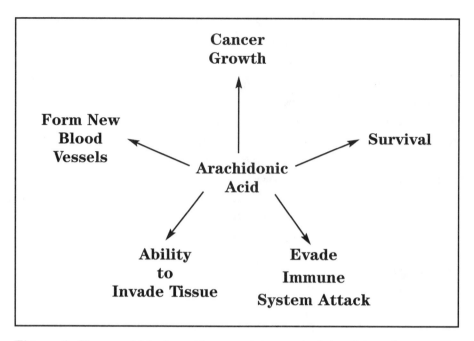

Figure 1. The arachidonic acid present in meat, dairy fat, and egg yolks stimulates prostate cancer survival, growth, invasion, and new blood vessel formation (angiogenesis).

experiments, such as rats and mice, this conversion is so efficient that a diet rich in plant oils will support high levels of arachidonic acid. This is not the case for humans — we are much less efficient in converting linoleic acid to arachidonic acid.

The implications of this research for prostate cancer treatment are potentially profound. If you switch to a vegan diet, you will significantly reduce arachidonic acid levels in your blood. If you take the additional step of switching to a low fat vegan diet, especially one that limits linoleic acid, you will reduce arachidonic acid levels to a greater extent. As you will see, lowering your arachidonic acid level may be prudent because it deprives your cancer of powerful hormones able to stimulate cancer growth and invasion.

Dietary arachidonic acid does not cause any acute side effects. The typical American ingests about 100 milligrams of arachidonic acid each day. In clinical studies, people have tolerated five to ten times this amount for close to two months with no problems of any kind. It is only at a dose of 7,000 milligrams a day that acute side effects have been reported in humans. The serious problems appear to develop only after chronic ingestion and in the context of preexisting disease, such as cancer.

Some investigators have argued that a diet rich in meat, and thus arachidonic acid, should not be of concern because humans evolved eating a diet rich in wild animal meat. Because humans survived hundreds of thousands of years on this diet, we must be well adapted to it. While this idea is superficially attractive, the average life span of humans in primitive societies was typically under forty years. The diseases linked to high intake of animal fat, such as heart disease and cancer, are most common over the age of fifty, long after the majority of people would have died! Modern civilization has created an artificial situation effectively doubling the life span of humans, thereby exposing us to diseases we are evolutionarily ill equipped to handle.

Conversion to Powerful Hormones

There is evidence that arachidonic acid is able to directly stimulate the growth of some cancer cells. This does not appear to be the case for prostate cancer cells. Arachidonic acid must be converted to one of several powerful hormones. The family of hormones derived from arachidonic acid is called "eicosanoids." While this name may seem strange to you, its effects are very much a part of daily life. For example, aspirin is able to relieve pain because it blocks the conversion of arachidonic acid to an eicosanoid, prostaglandin E2 or PGE2 that causes pain. Figure 2 shows the major eicosanoids that can be made from arachidonic acid. Of these, 5-HETE, 12-HETE, and PGE2 are known to be made by prostate cancer cells and to play a role in the growth and spread of this disease.

Arachidonic Acid and the Immune System

In past few years we have witnessed a dramatic expansion in our understanding of how the immune system acts to suppress the development of cancer. There are two cells critical to this process, the natural killer cells and the cytotoxic T cells. Both of these cells physically attach to and then kill the cancer cells.

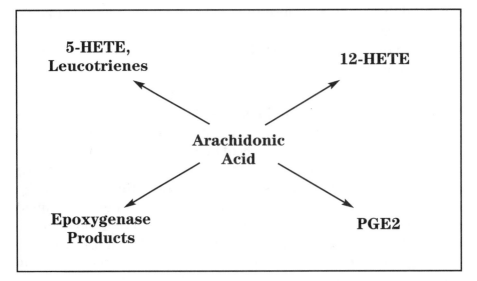

Figure 2. Arachidonic acid is converted to a wide range of powerful hormones. Human prostate cells are known to make PGE2, 5-HETE and 12-HETE.

This process requires that the immune cell find and then recognize the cancer cells.

In men over the age of 50, immune cells are common throughout the normal prostate tissue. If you examine radical prostatectomy specimens, you will find that immune cells are uncommon in prostate cancers of Gleason grades of 7 or higher. Some process has eliminated the immune cells from the higher-grade prostate cancers and the area immediately surrounding the cancer.

Arachidonic acid can be converted to a chemical PGE2. We have known for a long time that human prostate cancer cells produce PGE2 from arachidonic acid. In radical prostatectomy specimens, the cancer produced ten times as much PGE2 as the surrounding normal prostate tissue! PGE2 is very toxic to both natural killer cells and cytotoxic T cells and is one potential mechanism by which prostate cancer defeats the immune system.

Arachidonic Acid and Cancer Cell Invasion

Many patients do not have a clear understanding of how cancer cells spread. The cancer does not just get bigger and bigger until it breaks out of the prostate gland. Chunks of cancer do not break off into the blood stream and float about like a tree branch that falls into a river. Cancer cells actively invade! It is amazing to watch a time-lapse video of cancer cells in motion. They send out small extensions like tentacles. If these "tentacles" find places of attachment, they then pull the rest of the cancer cells along. When cancer cells come to a barrier blocking their movement, they are capable of "eating" their way through most obstacles. They then pull themselves through the hole they have created.

Cancer cells do not move about in a "blind" fashion. They are able to sense the presence of other cells and tissues because these cells and tissues send out chemical messages. In the case of human prostate cancer cells, they are attracted to bone cells. Figure 3 describes a common laboratory experiment that illustrates the power of this process. The essential apparatus is a tube that is separated into upper and lower portions by a plate. This plate has holes in it about a quarter the size of the cancer cells. The cancer cells are placed in the upper portion of the well. In the lower portion of the well, we place a fluid in which bone marrow cells have grown. Within a few minutes, the cancer cells will "sense" the presence of the bone marrow cells and move toward the lower well. In the process, they will eat their way through any normal tissue that is in the way, squeeze themselves through the small holes, and drop into the lower well.

Arachidonic acid markedly stimulates the ability of human prostate cancer cells to move and invade. This process is facilitated by the conversion of arachidonic acid to a substance called 12-HETE. Inhibitors of 12-HETE formation are remarkably effective at arresting the movement of human prostate cancer cells.

Tumor Blood Vessel Formation and 12-HETE

As cancers grow, they need more oxygen and food. They also generate more waste products that must be removed. The only way a cancer can satisfy these needs is to increase the size and number of blood vessels that supply the cancer. The process of new blood vessel formation is called angiogenesis (Figure 4).

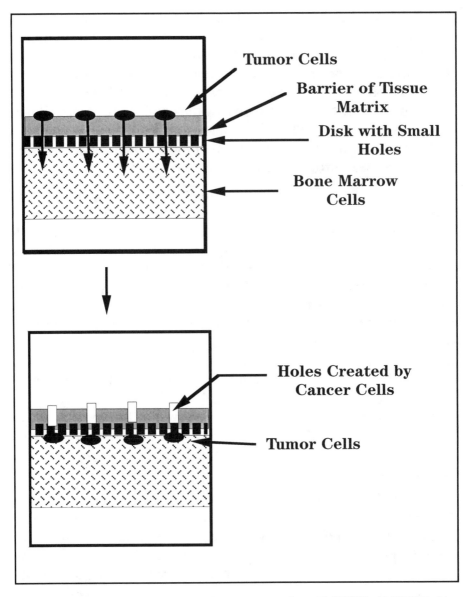

Figure 3. When arachidonic acid is converted to 12-HETE, 12-HETE then increases the ability of the cancer cells to invade. In the laboratory, this is measured using a plate with small holes in it. On top of this plate, we place a barrier made-up of the same material that lines blood vessels. The prostate cancer cells are placed on top of this barrier. Under the influence of 12-HETE, these cancer cells eat their way through the barrier and squeeze through the small holes. This test shows that this product of arachidonic acid stimulates the cancer cells to move, to eat through barriers, and to distort their shape if they need to reach their goal.

The pioneer in this research area is Dr. Judah Folkman. One of Dr. Folkman's most important observations is that new blood vessel formation is not a very active process in healthy adults. In a patient with cancer, nearly all of the new blood vessel formation happens in the cancer. Thus, treatments that block new blood vessel formation may prevent cancer growth while causing little or no side effects for the patient. Because of this work, the search for drugs able to block new blood vessel formation has become one of the "hot" areas of biotechnology. In the past year, two promising drugs, angiostatin and endostatin, were featured in articles in the New York Times, Newsweek, and Time.

Recently, Dr. Kenneth Honn from Wayne State Medical School in Detroit published an important paper linking conversion of arachidonic acid to 12-HETE in angiogenesis required for the growth of human prostate cancer. Dr. Honn and his colleagues first showed that simply adding 12-HETE to prostate cancer cells

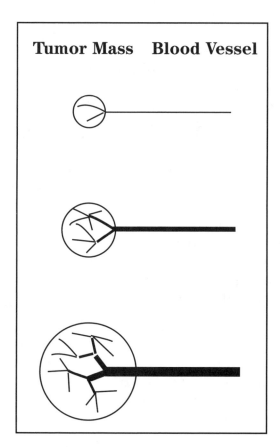

Tumor Mass Blood Vessel

Figure 4. As a cancer mass grows larger, it must form new blood vessels to feed the larger cancer. In medicine, we call a large mass of cancer cells a malignant tumor. This process of new blood vessel formation is stimulated by 12-HETE.

did not increase the growth rate of these cells. They then inserted additional copies of the gene controlling 12-HETE formation into these human prostate cancer cells. The original cancer cells and those engineered to make large amounts of 12-HETE were injected into mice. The cancers making increased amounts of 12-HETE grew much more rapidly. When the cancers were examined under the microscope, those making large amounts of 12-HETE also had more blood vessels.

In a separate study, Dr. Honn and his colleagues examined radical prostatectomy specimens to see which cancers had the capacity to make 12-HETE and which did not. They found that patients with tumors able to make 12-HETE were much more likely to develop metastatic prostate cancer after radical prostatectomy. Given the ability of 12-HETE to foster cancer cell invasion and new blood vessel formation these findings are hardly surprising.

Tumor Growth, Survival, and 5-HETE

Beginning in the mid 1980's, a series of investigators reported that the addition of arachidonic acid stimulated the growth of prostate cancer cells. None of these investigators was able to determine how arachidonic acid managed to increase the growth of these cancer cells.

In 1995, a young investigator in Dr. Myers' laboratory, Jagat Ghosh, took on this problem. He was able to confirm that arachidonic acid stimulated the growth of both hormone-sensitive and hormone-independent human prostate cancer cells. Most cancer cells require a rich broth full of nutrients to grow. If cancer cells are placed in just salt water, they stop growing and many will die in a day or two. He found that human prostate cancer cells needed only salt water and arachidonic acid to be able to survive and grow. He found that arachidonic acid had to be converted to 5-HETE to stimulate the growth of prostate cancer cells.

When we completely block the formation of 5-HETE, all human prostate cancer cell lines that we have been able to test stop growing and die within a few hours. Human prostate cancer cells contain a suicide program waiting to be activated. Hormonal therapy, radiation therapy, and chemotherapy treatments for prostate cancer work by activating this suicide program. None of these treatments cause cancer cell death as rapidly as is seen after we block 5-HETE formation.

The pathway by which arachidonic acid is converted to 5-HETE plays a major role in other diseases, including asthma, rheumatoid arthritis, and psoriasis. Ironically, this pathway does not seem to be necessary for the health of humans or other mammals. Genetic engineering has been used to produce mice that make no 5-HETE. These mice bear offspring that are normal and mature into normal adults. Therefore, a drug that blocks the formation of 5-HETE might be effective against prostate cancer and have few side effects.

Summary:

Arachidonic acid is able to increase new blood vessel formation, enhance invasiveness, speed growth and block the death of prostate cancer cells (Figure 5). The major dietary

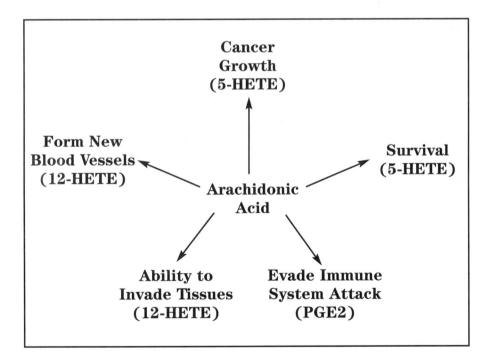

Figure 5. We showed that arachidonic acid is converted to a series of powerful hormones that promote the advance of prostate cancer. This figure summarizes these relationships.

sources of this fatty acid are meat, dairy fat and egg yolks and its presence provides a reasonable explanation for the fact that these foods appear to enhance the risk of metastatic prostate cancer.

References:

The first reference discusses the importance of essential fatty acids in the development of the human fetus.

L. Zhang. "The effects of essential fatty acids preparation in the treatment of intrauterine growth retardation" American Journal of Perinatology 14: 535-537, 1997.

The second reference discusses the importance of essential fatty acids in adults who must be fed by injection into their veins.

E. A. Mascioli, et al. "Essential fatty acid deficiency and home total parenteral nutrition patients" Nutrition 12: 245-249, 1996.

E. Giovannucci, et al. "A Prospective Study of Dietary Fat and Risk of Prostate Cancer" Journal of the National Cancer Institute 85: 1571-1579, 1993.

P. Gann, et al. "Prospective Study of Plasma Fatty Acids and Risk of Prostate Cancer" Journal of the National Cancer Institute 86: 281-286, 1994.

S.D. Phinney, et al. "Reduced Arachidonate in Serum Phospholipids and Cholesteryl Esters Associated with Vegetarian Diets" American Journal of Clinical Nutrition 51: 385-392, 1990.

This is the lead article in an entire issue of the journal, Lipids, devoted to understanding the acute consequences of elevated arachidonic acid intake.

G.J. Nelson, et al. "A Human Dietary Arachidonic Acid Supplementation Study Conducted in a Metabolic Research Unit: Rationale and Design" Lipids 32: 415-420, 1997.

The next paper examined the impact of very high doses of arachidonic acid. The study was terminated early because of potentially serious side effects.

H. W. Seyberth, et al. "Increased Arachidonate in Lipids After Administration to Man" Clinical Pharmacology and Therapeutics 18: 521-529, 1975.

The next paper discusses the potential importance of arachidonic acid in humans living in primitive societies.

A.J. Sinclair, et al. "The Significance of Arachidonic Acid in Hunter-Gatherer Diets: Implications for the Contemporary Western Diet" Journal of Food Lipids 1: 143-157, 1993.

The following papers cover the role of various arachidonic acid products in the biology of prostate cancer.

B. Liu, et al. "12(S)-HETE enhancement of prostate tumor cell invasion: selective role of PKC alpha" Journal of the National Cancer Institute 86: 1145-1151, 1994.

K. V. Honn, et al. "Tumor cell-derived 12 (S)-HETE induces microvascular endothelial cell retraction" Cancer Research 54: 565-574, 1994.

X. Gao, A. T. Porter and K.V. Honn. "Involvement of the multiple tumor suppressor genes and 12-Lipoxygenase in Human Prostate Cancer: therapeutic implications" Advances in Experimental Medicine and Biology 407: 41-53, 1997.

K.V. Honn, et al. "12-Lipoxygenase and 12(S)-HETE: role in cancer metastasis" Cancer Metastasis Review 13: 365-396, 1994.

N. Weidner, et al. "Tumor angiogenesis correlates with metastasis in invasive prostate carcinoma" American Journal of Pathology 143: 401-409, 1993.

D.G. Tang, et al. "12(S)-HETE is a mitogenic factor for microvascular endothelial cells: its potential role in angiogenesis" Biochemical Biophysical Research Communication 211: 462-468, 1995.

D. Nie, et al. "Platelet-type 12-lipoxygenase in a human prostate carcinoma stimulates angiogenesis and tumor growth" Cancer Research 58:4047-4051, 1998.

J. Ghosh and Charles Myers. "Arachidonic Acid Stimulates Prostate Cancer Cell Growth: Critical Role of 5-Lipoxygenase" Biochemical and Biophysical Research Communications 235: 418-423, 1997.

J. Ghosh and Charles Myers. "Inhibition of arachidonate-lipoxygenase triggers massive apoptosis in human prostate cancer cells" Proceedings of the National Academy of Sciences 95: 13182-13187, 1998.

Antioxidants

Supplements containing antioxidants are very popular. They have been recommended for the prevention of heart disease, stroke, aging, and cancer. In the case of prostate cancer, there is strong evidence that antioxidants can decrease the number of deaths from this disease. It is important for you to realize that there are major differences in how the various antioxidants operate.

What are antioxidants and why are they important? Oxygen is obviously a requirement for human life. It may seem odd to you that oxygen is a double-edged sword capable of causing tissue injury and even death! The air we breathe is only 20% oxygen – much of the rest is nitrogen. If you were forced to breathe 100% oxygen for a prolonged period of time, it would cause enough lung damage to kill you. Oxygen is one of those things in life that is good only in moderation.

Why is oxygen dangerous? Nearly all of the tissues in your body can convert oxygen to hydrogen peroxide. In turn, hydrogen peroxide can trigger a complex series of events capable of causing enormous damage and even death of any tissue in your body. This process involves the formation of free radicals, chemical compounds so reactive that they can destroy life in a fraction of a second.

When life on earth started, there was little or no oxygen in the air. Early life forms evolved to live in the absence of oxygen. A key event in the march of life was the appearance of the first plants, single cell algae. Plants capture the energy of sunlight and convert it into chemical energy that they then use to live and grow. As a by-product of this process, oxygen is released.

With the appearance of algae, the world experienced its first environmental disaster: rapidly increasing oxygen levels killed large numbers of other life forms that were completely unprepared to defend themselves against the hydrogen peroxide formed from oxygen. The major problem with oxygen is that it can be converted to hydrogen peroxide. Hydrogen peroxide can cause damage or kill living organisms because it can be converted into very reactive chemicals called free radicals. It was in the wake of this environmental disaster that organisms emerged capable of defending themselves against oxygen. These new life forms came to dominate the earth and became ancestors of all animal life on the planet, including humans.

What were the innovations that allowed the new life forms to survive in the presence of oxygen? These cells first learned how to convert hydrogen peroxide and other dangerous forms of oxygen into water. A second key step involved producing chemicals that inactivate any free radicals that form. The third step involved learning how to repair the damage caused by hydrogen peroxide and free radicals. All useful antioxidants work by aiding the conversion of hydrogen peroxide to water, inactivating free radicals, or repairing the damage oxygen causes.

As with other animals, human tissues protect themselves against damage by hydrogen peroxide and other reactive oxygen compounds. This process is not 100% effective and even under normal conditions oxygen damage to tissues accumulate as we age. Additionally, nutritional deficiencies can disable the defenses against hydrogen peroxide. As we will see, the latter appears to play a major role in the development of prostate cancer.

Why should hydrogen peroxide and reactive free radicals play a role in the development of prostate cancer? Chemicals that damage the genetic material (DNA) in cells cause cancer. This damage alters the function of those genes important in the regulation of cell multiplication, resulting in the uncontrolled growth characteristic of cancer. These reactive oxygen compounds are well known to cause DNA damage and to promote the development of cancer.

There is now evidence linking the creation of hydrogen peroxide with prostate cancer. The male sex hormones, testosterone and dihydrotestosterone, are required for the development of prostate cancer in men. Furthermore, exposure to high concentrations of these androgens increases the risk of prostate cancer. The addition of androgens to prostate cells triggers the production of hydrogen peroxide. Furthermore, prostate cancer cells either lack completely, or have reduced levels, of several proteins important in reducing the toxicity of oxygen. These observations provide a direct link between factors known to foster the development of prostate cancer and the production of hydrogen peroxide.

References:

M.O. Ripple, et al. "Provident-antioxidant shift induced by androgen treatment of human prostate carcinoma cells" Journal of the National Cancer Institute 89: 40-48, 1997.

A.M. Baker, et al. "Expression of antioxidant enzymes in human prostatic adenocarcinoma" Prostate 32: 229-233, 1997.

W.H. Lee, et al. "Cytidine methylation of regulatory sequences near the pi-class glutathione S-transferase gene accompanies human prostatic carcinogenesis" Proceedings of the National Academy of Sciences 91: 11733-11737, 1994.

Selenium

A protein called glutathione peroxidase is an important part of the body's normal defense against hydrogen peroxide. This protein is one of the most effective means available for converting hydrogen peroxide to water. Selenium is an essential part of this protein and it contains more than 95% of the selenium in your body. Without selenium, the tissues in your body are destroyed by hydrogen peroxide. For humans and most other mammals, the first tissue to fail is the heart.

The Side Effects of Selenium

It may seem strange to begin this section with a discussion of the toxic side effects of selenium. However, this has a historical rationale because selenium first came to attention of the medical profession because of the problems caused by high intake of selenium. It was only later that the beneficial effects of selenium were documented. The perception of selenium as dangerous remains common in the medical and nutritional communities. As you will see, selenium actually has a safety margin similar to that of calcium and other common nutrients.

Selenium concentrates in your skin and hair. As a result, a mild overdose of selenium will make your hair dry and brittle (see Table 1). Your nails will also become brittle, thickened and may develop ridges. At somewhat higher doses, your nails will break and drop off. You will also develop red swollen skin lesions that can evolve into blisters. These skin lesions usually cause severe itching. Finally, very high doses will cause brain damage and death.

We also need to emphasize that in the Northern Great Plains of the United States, the soil and water are rich in selenium. Farm animals in this region can suffer from "alkali disease" or "blind staggers" if they graze on plants that accumulate selenium.

Astralagus is an herbal product that many prostate cancer patients are taking. There are about 300 Astralagus species in the Western United States. Of these, 25 are known to be active accumulators of selenium. We do not know whether the medicinal Astralagus species are selenium accumulators.

Therefore, we urge you to be cautious about taking herbal products containing astralagus and selenium at the same time.

Selenium is not the only nutrient that is dangerous if you take too much. Both vitamins A and D can be lethal. Even calcium can cause serious injury or death if you ingest too much. As a general principle, we recommend that you carefully investigate the safety of taking more than the recommended daily dose of any vitamin or mineral. Remember, even table salt can kill you if you eat too much of it.

Despite these toxic side effects, Table 1 shows there is a fairly large margin of safety between selenium doses implicated in cancer prevention and those that cause toxicity.

Table 1. Biological effects of selenium.

Daily Dose (mcg per day):	Biological Effects:
Below 10	Severe deficiency will develop
15-30	Minimum daily dose
40-50	Adequate daily intake
200	For selenium deficient areas
400	Suggested maximum from natural diet
600	Maximum safe dietary dose
900	Mild side effects may develop
1,500-2,000	Mild to moderate side effects in most people
more than 4,000	Loss of hair and nails, brain damage

Selenium Is An Essential Nutrient

In the United States, the Food and Nutrition Board of the National Academy of Sciences set the Recommended Dietary Allowances (RDA). The process by which this Board develops its recommendations is quite conservative, with a heavy emphasis on safety and ample proof that a nutrient is truly necessary. Often, the dose selected is quite low. For example, the RDA for vitamin E in men is only 10 International Units!

After due deliberation, the Food and Nutrition Board officially recognized the role of selenium in human nutrition and has assigned a RDA for this mineral. The development of recommendations for selenium was beset by controversy. The early literature on selenium largely focused on its toxicity and this created a negative image that delayed recognition of its key role in human health. As we have just pointed out, the toxicity of this mineral has been over emphasized. In a sense, it is a tribute to the strength of the evidence supporting the importance of selenium that these difficulties were surmounted. The selenium RDA for adults ranges from 60-75 mcg, depending on body size.

The World Health Organization (WHO) also examined the daily selenium intake necessary to preserve health. They concluded that 16-21 mcgs were required to protect against severe deficiency side effects such as sudden death. They concluded that doses of 30 to 40 mcgs were sufficient to provide an adequate safety margin. These values were set with an eye toward general health issues and not with the goal of cancer prevention.

The major point of this discussion is to show that the role of selenium in human nutrition has been carefully reviewed. It has been determined that selenium is an essential nutrient.

Geography Of Selenium Deficiency

In the United States, areas with low selenium levels in soil and forage crops include much of the Atlantic Coastal Plain, Pennsylvania, Ohio, the Upper Mississippi river valley, the eastern two thirds of Washington and Oregon as well as Northern California. In Virginia, were we live, selenium deficiency in forage crops is a well-known agricultural problem, and farm animals are routinely given selenium supplements.

Outside the United States, low selenium levels have been documented in New Zealand, Finland and in parts of China. In each of these areas, programs of selenium supplementation of soils, animal feed or humans have been established. A recent article in the journal Lancet documented a recent, rather dramatic decline in selenium intake in Great Britain and other parts of Western Europe with serious potential health implications.

What causes selenium depletion of soils? When soils are moist and acid, selenium undergoes conversion to hydrogen selenide, a gas that can dissolve in water. Excess rain can leach hydrogen selenide from the soils. If the soils are plowed, hydrogen selenide readily escapes into the air. Acid rain and frequent plowing of soil may well accelerate this process.

Selenium And Cancer Prevention

The National Cancer Institute compiles detailed information on cancer death rates in various geographic regions of the United States. Because of its importance for animal husbandry, information was also available from the US Department of Agriculture on soil selenium levels throughout much of this country. When these two lists were compared, cancer deaths were much higher in those areas low in soil selenium. These findings suggested that higher levels of selenium played an important role in preventing cancer, presumably by eliminating hydrogen peroxide and the damage it can cause.

The importance of selenium in cancer prevention has received support from several recent studies. In the December, 1996, issue of the Journal of the American Medical Association, Clark, et al., reported the results of a clinical trial in which half of the people received 200 mcg of selenium-containing yeast a day and the other half were left on their normal diet. The results were quite striking: the incidence of all cancers were reduced by more than 50% and prostate cancer by more than 60%. For those men with initial PSA values in the normal range, selenium supplementation reduced the risk of prostate cancer by 74%. Several other investigators have confirmed a link between selenium and the risk of prostate cancer, although none of these other trials are randomized controlled clinical trials.

The study by Dr. Clark was conducted with people from the Mid Atlantic region, an area where the soil was known to be selenium deficient. The dose of selenium used, 200 mcgs, was much higher than the RDA, but side effects were not noted during the conduct of this trial, indicating that this higher dose is well tolerated by people living in an area where soils are selenium deficient. We think that the evidence available suggests that the current RDA for selenium may be too low for those living in these areas and a dose of 200 mcg a day may be more appropriate.

As we mentioned, there are areas of the country where soil selenium is adequate or even high. Most nutrition experts consider a dose of 200 mcg a day to be too high for people living in areas with high selenium soils, such as the Northern Great Plains. In fact, people in these regions may need no selenium supplementation. If you are not sure of the situation in your area, we know of two solutions. One is to have your blood selenium measured. At the University of Virginia there is a blood test available. You may want to check with the major hospitals in your area. The second solution is to ask your county agricultural extension agent or, failing that, farmers or veterinarians in your region whether selenium is needed for the health of the animals.

The clinical trial we just discussed was designed to study the role of selenium in cancer prevention. Is selenium of value if you already have prostate cancer? Addition of selenium has been shown to kill cancer cells in the laboratory. The concentrations required appeared similar to levels found in people who live in areas with high soil selenium. Dr. Clark is currently conducting a clinical trial testing the value of high doses of selenium in the treatment of prostate cancer.

Should you take selenium? Selenium is an essential nutrient with a recommended daily allowance. If you live in an area with selenium deficient soils, we think you would be prudent to take it. Furthermore, the dose of 200 mcgs appears to be both effective and safe.

When you go to the health food store to purchase selenium, you will most likely find a bewildering range of choices. Dr. Clark's trial used selenium-yeast and this fact has made this form our first choice. Selenomethinonine is another form you may encounter. A majority of the selenium in the yeast preparation is in the form of selenomethinonine and this form appears to be appropriate. You may find sodium selenate or selenite. We do not recommend either of these as we have major reservations about how well either of these will be absorbed by your gut.

References:

The first paper is an early review by Dr. Clark that summarized the literature on the link between the geographic distribution of selenium and risk of cancer.

L.C. Clark, et al. "Selenium in forage crops and cancer mortality in U.S." Archives of Environmental Health 46: 37-42, 1991.

The next two papers report the results of Dr. Clark's large randomized controlled trials.

L.C. Clark, et al. "Effects of Selenium Supplementation for Cancer Prevention in Patients with Carcinoma of the Skin: A Randomized Controlled Trial" Journal of the American Medical Society 276:1957-1963, 1996.

L.C. Clark, et al. "Decreased Incidence of Prostate Cancer with Selenium Supplementation – Results of a Double-Blind Cancer Prevention Trial" British Journal of Urology 81: 730-734, 1998.

The next paper summarizes the World Health Organization's evaluation of selenium requirements.

O.A. Levander. "Selenium requirements as discussed in the 1996 joint FAO/IAEA/WHO expert consultation on trace elements in human nutrition" Biochemical & Environmental Sciences 10: 214-219, 1997.

The next paper provides information on the link between selenium and cancer in Finland.

P. Kneckt, et al. "Serum Selenium and subsequent risk of cancer among Finnish men and women" Journal of the National Cancer Institute 82: 864-868, 1990.

The next two papers describe a direct effect of selenium on cancer cells in the laboratory.

C. Rodman, et al. "Inhibitory Effect of Selenomethinonine on the Growth of Three Selected Human Tumor Cell Lines" Cancer Letters 125: 103-110, 1998.

D.Y. Cho, et al. "Induction of apoptosis by selenite and selenodiglutathione in HL-60 cells" Biochemistry & Molecular Biology International 47: 781-793, 1999.

The next two papers are clinical trials suggesting other health benefits that might result from selenium supplementation.

F. Girodon, et al. "Impact of trace elements and vitamin supplementation on immunity and infections in institutionalized elderly patients – A randomized controlled trial" Archives of Internal Medicine 159: 748-754, 1999.

A. Campa, et al. "Mortality risk in selenium-deficient HIV-positive children" Journal of Acquired Immune Deficiency Syndromes & Human Retrovirology 20: 508-513, 1999.

We recommend these two recent reviews, because they are fascinating reading and an excellent guide to the literature on selenium safety.

J. Spallholz. "On the nature of selenium toxicity and carcinostatic activity" Free Radical Biology and Medicine 17: 45-64, 1994.

P. Whanger, et al. "Metabolism of subtoxic levels of selenium in animals and humans" Annals of Clinical and Laboratory Science 26: 99-113, 1996.

Vitamin E

Vitamin E dissolves in fat, not water. In the body, it is found in your fatty tissues and in globules of fat that are present in the blood. A fatty layer called the cell membrane surrounds each cell and vitamin E is present in that membrane as well. Vitamin E only acts as an antioxidant for the fatty material at these sites.

Another aspect of vitamin E is the manner in which it acts as an antioxidant. Oxygen free radicals attack vitamin E and both parties are destroyed in the interaction. In other words, vitamin E is sacrificed so that free radical damage to normal tissues may be prevented. The greater the number of oxygen radicals being produced, the greater the amount of vitamin E that will be needed.

We now have a randomized controlled clinical trial that documents the value of vitamin E in men. In this study, 23,000 Finnish men were randomly assigned to four groups: vitamin E alone, beta-carotene alone, both vitamin E and beta-carotene, and no supplement. At the time the article was published, the men had been on the study for 5 to 8 years. The men on vitamin E alone had 32% fewer cases of prostate cancer and 41% fewer deaths from this disease.

The impact of vitamin E became apparent after the men were on vitamin E for only two years. These findings cannot be due to prevention of prostate cancer. To have an effect on the number of prostate cancer deaths within 2 years, vitamin E must be able to suppress the growth and spread of prostate cancer. Furthermore, vitamin E would have to have had an effect on the more aggressive forms of this cancer.

The dose of vitamin E used in this study was actually quite low. Doses of Vitamin E are expressed as either International

Units or milligrams. One milligram of alpha-tocopherol (vitamin E) equals one International Unit. Most drug and grocery stores carry vitamin E capsules of 200 to 1,000 International Units. In this study, the dose of vitamin E was 50 International Units. A low dose is very safe and costs only about 10 cents a day.

If 50 International Units were active, why not take more? As with any vitamin or mineral, there are risks with too much vitamin E. At least one study suggested that doses higher than 400 International Units might suppress immune function. Doses above 1,000 International Units have been associated with an increased risk of bleeding.

There are several caveats worth mentioning. This is just one randomized controlled study, although a very large one and it would be nice to see another study confirm these results. Also, this study was originally designed to examine the impact of vitamin E on smokers. It is possible that vitamin E only prevents prostate cancer in smokers, but we do not think that likely. Finally, this study was conducted in Finland, an area with low selenium levels, and it is possible that the impact of vitamin E may be less impressive in men with adequate selenium intake. Thus, while evidence strongly suggests that vitamin E is valuable in preventing prostate cancer, this has not been proven. We do not think these concerns should prevent you from taking vitamin E in doses that range from 200 to 400 International Units. Vitamin E in this dose range is safe, inexpensive and has other health benefits. In other words, the risk is small and the potential benefit is large.

Green Tea Polyphenols

We remember when we first heard about the possible anticancer activities of green tea. It seemed almost beyond belief that something so plain, so simple, could be of value. Yet the evidence is becoming more and more impressive. Green tea has attracted the scientific community's attention and interesting work is being done on the mechanism by which green tea reduces the risk of cancer.

Green tea is rich in compounds called polyphenols that are potent antioxidants. This antioxidant activity may account for green tea's ability to lessen sun damage and to prevent the action of many cancer-causing chemicals.

It is apparent that green tea can not only prevent cancer, but is able to stop the growth or even kill human cancer cells. This ability was documented in human breast, lung, colon, pancreatic, and prostate cancers.

The contents of green tea have been carefully examined to determine the chemical in the tea responsible for the anticancer activity. There seems to be a growing consensus that most of the useful activity is caused by a polyphenol called epigallocatechin gallate or EGCG. This compound caused the rapid shrinkage of human prostate cancers growing in mice.

Cancer cells increase in number by doubling, one cell becomes two, two become four, four become eight, and so on. Green tea appears to halt the growth of cancer cells by preventing one cancer cell from splitting into two cells. This is the same point where two other drugs active against prostate cancer, taxol and vinblastine, also work. In addition, cells arrested at this point are unusually sensitive to radiation therapy. We think it would be interesting to test whether green tea extracts improve the results of radiation therapy.

At higher concentrations, equivalent to someone drinking more than 10 cups of tea per day, ECGC causes prostate and other cancer cells to commit suicide. In the case of prostate cancer, ECGC is able to kill the human prostate cancer cell line, DU145. This is the most aggressive and most therapy-resistant of any human prostate cancer cell line available.

EGCG and other green tea polyphenols are sensitive to light and air. These polyphenols are much more stable in the presence of acid and vitamin C. EGCG is oxidized on exposure to air and vitamin C prevents this. It would seem prudent to add a little lemon juice to the tea as it is being brewed: the citric acid in the juice will make the tea acidic and the juice is rich in vitamin C. The tea should either be drunk soon after it has been made or chilled rapidly to make an iced tea.

The amount of EGCG found in green tea appears to be effective as a cancer prevention agent. The amount needed to stop the growth of cancer cells or to cause the cancer to shrink rapidly in mice is much larger than that associated with green tea consumption. Green tea appears to be very safe with the only significant side effects coming from its caffeine content. The large doses required to cause arrest or death of tumor growth would also involve a large dose of caffeine. Green tea extracts allow larger doses to be taken and are available with reduced caffeine content or caffeine-free. These are available in many health food stores. Doses as high as a gram (1,000 milligrams) a day have been taken with no reported side effects.

Quercetin

Quercetin, a chemical found in plants, has a wide range of desirable attributes. It is a powerful antioxidant shown to prevent damage caused by hydrogen peroxide. It prevents oxidation of fats in the blood, may have a role in slowing or preventing heart disease, and has a number of useful antitumor activities.

Bcl2 is a protein found in many cancer cells that allows cancer cells to escape death during radiation therapy, chemotherapy, and hormonal therapy by producing abnormally large amounts of this protein. Quercitin reduces the amount of bcl2 in cells.

When cancer cells double, they do so by building a device called the mitotic spindle that then pulls and divides the cell into two daughter cells. Some of our most useful cancer drugs, such as taxol, vinblastine, and estramustine (Emcyt) are active anticancer drugs because they prevent the mitotic spindle from functioning. Quercetin also blocks the assembly of the mitotic spindle, but without any of the toxicity caused by these chemotherapy drugs.

Cancer cells become particularly sensitive to radiation therapy when their ability to form a mitotic spindle is blocked. Clinical trials have already demonstrated that taxol and estramustine interact favorably with radiation therapy. As with these other inhibitors of mitotic spindle formation, Quercetin also enhances the activity of radiation therapy in the laboratory.

Quercetin is present in many fruits and vegetables. Rich sources include raspberries, strawberries, red wine, broccoli, and chocolate. Red and yellow onions are particularly rich sources, while white onions have low levels of this compound. Many of the recipes in this book include foods rich in Quercetin.

References:

J. Vanrijn and J. Vandenberg. "Flavonoids as Enhancers of X-ray-induced Cell Damage in Hepatoma Cells" Clinical Cancer Research 3: 1775-1779, 1997.

T. Takagi, et al. "Quercetin, a flavonol, promotes disassembly of microtubules in prostate cancer cells: Possible mechanism of its antitumor activity" Acta Histochemica et Cytochemica 31: 435-445, 1998.

S.C. Lee, et al. "Bioflavonoids commonly and potentially induce tyrosine dephosphorylation/Inactivation of Oncogenic Proline-Directed Protein Kinase FA in Human Prostate Carcinoma Cells" Anticancer Research 18:1117-1121, 1998.

D. Xiao, et al. "Quercetin Down-regulated BCL-2 Gene Expression in Human Leukemia HL-60 Cells" Acta Pharmacologica Sinica 19: 551-553, 1998.

M. Paolini. "On the Cancer Chemoprevention Potential of Dietary Bio-flavonoids" Mutagenesis 13: 535-536, 1998.

C. A. Musonda and J. K. Chipman. "Quercetin inhibits Hydrogen Peroxide-induced NF-Kappa-B DNA Binding Activity and DNA Damage in HepG2 Cells" Carcinogenesis 19: 1583-1589, 1998.

Carotenoids

Beta-carotene is the orange pigment found in many orange vegetables, such as carrots and sweet potatoes. It is a member of a large group of plant pigments called the carotenoids, with colors ranging from yellow through orange to red. Examples include the yellow pigment in marigolds, as well as the red color in tomatoes, lycopene.

When light strikes a leaf, part of the energy is used in photosynthesis to make sugars. The remaining unused energy is capable of rapidly destroying the leaf. The carotenoids, including beta-carotene, are critical in preventing the destructive side effects of photosynthesis. In some of these reactions, the carotenoids act as powerful antioxidants, a factor that may be important in their ability to prevent some forms of cancer in people.

You do not see these pigments normally because the green of the chlorophyll hides the carotenoids. In autumn the chlorophyll disappears, the carotenoids are revealed and make their contribution to the beautiful fall foliage as the major source of the yellow, orange, and warm red tones.

In the human body, carotenoids can act as antioxidants. Of the common carotenoids, lycopene is the most active in blocking oxidative damage. Some of the carotenoids, such as beta-carotene, can be converted into vitamin A. Knowing the effect of beta-carotene and related compounds involves understanding their direct action and that of vitamin A.

The point of this discussion is that carotenoids can both give rise to vitamin A and act as antioxidants. Furthermore, while beta-carotene is a carotenoid that can be converted to vitamin A, there are other carotenoids, such as lycopene, that cannot.

Impact of Beta-Carotene and Vitamin A on Prostate Cancer

Most of the work on the impact of beta-carotene and vitamin A on prostate cancer were epidemiology studies. In this type of study, investigators record the diets and cancer status of a group of men. The investigators then look to see what items in the diet were more or less common in those patients who developed prostate cancer.

Most of these studies have shown little or no effect of either beta-carotene or vitamin A on prostate cancer. However, a small number have shown an increased risk of prostate cancer among men with a higher intake of these nutrients! We were skeptical about the negative results reported for prostate cancer because beta-carotene and vitamin A have impressive activity against a wide range of human cancers. Pharmaceutical companies have been quite active in searching for drugs based on the active form of vitamin A, retinoic acid.

All-trans-retinoic acid, a form of vitamin A, has revolutionized the treatment of certain leukemias. Another drug, fenretinide, has shown considerable promise in breast cancer prevention. Breast and prostate cancer have many similarities. Therefore it was logical to test fenretinide against prostate cancer and, indeed, laboratory studies showed that this drug had some promise against prostate cancer.

This led to a clinical trial by Kenneth Pienta of the University of Michigan. In this trial, twenty-two men with a PSA of greater than 4, but with a negative prostate biopsy, were placed on fenretinide. After six months, patients had a repeat biopsy of their prostate gland. Unexpectedly, 40% now had prostate cancer present in their biopsies! These results certainly suggest that fenretinide does not represent a revolutionary advance in the prevention of prostate cancer. It may well be that this drug actually increased the risk of prostate cancer.

This discussion has prepared you to appreciate the significance of a randomized controlled clinical trial. In the Finnish study (mentioned in the previous section on vitamin E), vitamin E and beta-carotene were compared with no treatment. The goal of this trial was to determine if either vitamin E or beta-carotene lessened the risk of lung cancer among cigarette smokers.

The study involved more than 20,000 male cigarette smokers from Finland. One quarter of the patients took nothing. A second quarter of the patients took 50 International Units of vitamin E. A third quarter took 20 mg of beta-carotene. The final quarter took both vitamin E and beta-carotene. The incidence of clinically significant prostate cancer (Stage II - IV) decreased by 40% in the men receiving vitamin E, but increased by 35% in the men receiving beta-carotene!

There are some reasons to be cautious about this study. First, the study involved smokers and we cannot be absolutely sure that similar results would be obtained in nonsmokers. Second, while the study involved more than 20,000 men, there were only 246 cases of prostate cancer, 192 of which were clinically significant. Furthermore, there were only 62 prostate cancer deaths. The conclusions about beta-carotene involve an increase in clinically significant prostate cancers from 81 cases among the men not taking beta-carotene to 109 cases in those on this nutrient. The authors suggest that caution in interpreting the beta-carotene results is warranted.

What is our conclusion? We think there is no reason to take beta-carotene. It has not been shown to be either safe or effective in prostate cancer. Additionally, there is a very good chance that it may accelerate the development of this disease.

References:

O.P. Heinonen, et al. "Prostate Cancer and Supplementation with alpha-tocopherol and beta-carotene: incidence and mortality in a controlled trial" Journal of the National Cancer Institute 90: 440-446, 1998.

G. S. Omenn, et al. "Risk factors for lung cancer and for intervention effects n CARET, the beta carotene and retinol efficacy trial" Journal of the National Cancer Institute 88: 1550-1559, 1996.

Lycopene

Of the carotenoids, one of the most effective antioxidants, is lycopene. This pigment is red, instead of orange like beta-carotene. Tomatoes, red watermelon, and pink grapefruit are the three richest sources of lycopene and owe their red color to this pigment (see Table 2).

Table 2. Lycopene content of common foods.*

	Micrograms per gram:
Watermelon	23-72
Pink Guava	54
Pink Grapefruit	33
Papaya	20-53
Fresh Tomatoes	8.8-42
Cooked Tomatoes	37
Tomato Sauce	62
Tomato Paste	54-1,500
Tomato Soup (condensed)	80
Tomato Powder	1126-1265
Tomato Juice	50-116
Pizza Sauce	127
Ketchup	99-134

*(From Rao and Agarwal)

A diet high in tomato products and thus lycopene is associated with a reduced risk of prostate cancer. The greatest protection was associated with an intake of 10 or more servings of tomato products each week. In the tomato, lycopene is contained within small packets that are not readily broken down by the stomach and intestines. Cooking tomatoes significantly improves the ease with which you can absorb lycopene and is associated with the greatest impact on the risk of prostate cancer.

The simplest approach is to have an eight-ounce glass of tomato or V8 juice every morning with breakfast. For dinner, spaghetti, vegetarian chili or other tomato-based dishes can be used. With this diet, it is easy to eat at least 10 servings of tomatoes a week, a more pleasurable and less expensive way than taking lycopene capsules. If you prefer not to eat tomato products, you should take lycopene capsules. Currently, 5, 10, and 15 mg capsules are widely available. A recent study using 30 mg of lycopene in capsule form a day showed a decrease in the extent of prostate cancer at the time of radical prostatectomy. If you plan to take lycopene capsules, a dose of 30 mg may be a good starting point.

One interesting property of lycopene is that, once in the body, this pigment persists for several days. If you start to take lycopene, your blood and tissue levels will steadily increase each day for one week. This property means that it is not critical to take lycopene two to three times a day. Even missing one or two days may have only a modest impact on the concentration of lycopene in your tissues.

References:

E. Giovannucci, et al. "Intake of carotenoids and retinol in relation to risk of prostate cancer" Journal of the National Cancer Institute 87: 1767-1776, 1995.

P.H. Gann, et al. "Lower prostate cancer risk in men with elevated plasma lycopene levels: Results of a prospective analysis" Cancer Research 59: 12256-1230, 1999.

A.V. Rao, N Fleshner, and S. Agarwal. "Serum and tissue lycopene and bio-markers of oxidation in prostate cancer patients: A case-control study" Nutrition & Cancer – An International Journal 33: 159-164, 1999.

P.K. Mills, et al. "Cohort study of diet, lifestyle and prostate cancer in Adventist men" Cancer 64: 598-604, 1989.

E. Giovannucci, et al. "Tomatoes, tomato-based products, lycopene, and cancer: Review of the Epidemiologic Literature" Journal of the National Cancer Institute 91: 317-331, 1999.

A.V. Rao and S. Agarwal. "Role of lycopene as antioxidant carotinoid in the prevention of chronic diseases: A review" Nutrition Research 19: 305-323, 1999.

M.L. Nguyen and S.J. Schwartz. "Lycopene Stability During Food Processing" Proceedings of the Society for Experimental Biology & Medicine 218: 101-105, 1998.

M. Pastori, et al. "Lycopene in Association with Alpha-tocopherol inhibits at physiologic concentrations proliferation of prostate carcinoma cells" Biochemical & Biophysical Research Communications 250: 582-585, 1998.

M. Porrini, et al. "Absorption of Lycopene from single or daily portions of raw and processed tomato" British Journal of Nutrition 80: 353-361, 1998.

I. Paetau, et al. "Chronic ingestion of lycopene-rich tomato juice or lycopene supplements significantly increases plasma concentrations of lycopene and related tomato carotenoids in humans" American Journal of Clinical Nutrition 68: 1187-1195, 1998.

G.R. Beecher. "Nutrient Content of Tomatoes and Tomato Products" Proceedings of the Society for Experimental Biology and Medicine 218: 98-100, 1998.

T. Aburkao, et al. "Vitamin D3 and its metabolites in tomato, potato, eggplant and zucchini" Phytochemistry 49: 2497-2499, 1998.

Soybeans

Soybeans have dominated the diet of most Asian countries for thousands of years. Even in this country, the soybean is an important component of animal feed and of processed foods for human use.

The global importance of this legume is not an accident. The soybean produces 5 times as much protein per acre as wheat, 10 times as much as dairy cattle, and 25 times as much as beef cattle. As a legume, it manufactures its own nitrate fertilizer. Its roots travel deep into the soil and extract nutrients from subsoils where other plants can not. In the process, it improves the quality of the soil in which it is grown.

The soybean provides a source of high quality protein that is low in saturated fat and cholesterol-free. The intake of soy protein lowers the triglycerides, total amount of cholesterol, LDL or bad cholesterol without lowering the HDL or good cholesterol. The risk of heart disease is much lower in Asia, where soy is the dominant source of protein, compared with the USA and Europe, where animal products are the major source.

A diet rich in meat causes an increase in the loss of calcium into the urine. This means that men and women on a diet rich in meat are at an increased risk for osteoporosis. The increase in urinary calcium also increases the risk of kidney stones. A diet rich in soy protein causes much less loss of calcium into the urine and results in a lower risk of both osteoporosis and kidney stones.

Deaths from cancers of the breast, colon, and prostate are uncommon where soy intake is high. Soy's relation to prostate cancer is particularly interesting. The incidence of localized prostate cancer is relatively similar in the United States, Western Europe, and Asia. However, the risk of developing metastatic prostate cancer and dying from the disease is lower in Asia.

Phytoestrogens

Problems commonly associated with menopause, such as hot flashes and osteoporosis, are less common and less severe in women living in Asia. Soybeans contain a family of chemicals called isoflavones that act like the female sex hormone estrogen. They are also called phyto-estrogens: the prefix phyto- means "from plants". Dietary phytoestrogens found in soy may partially replace the loss of estrogen characteristic of menopause.

Estrogen and estrogen-like drugs have long been used to treat prostate cancer. In men, a hormone (LH), released by a portion of the brain stimulates testosterone production by the testes. Estrogen turns off the production of LH and thus testosterone. The result is a medical castration. Many have speculated that soy phytoestrogens reduce the risk of prostate cancer because they act like estrogen and lower the production of LH and thus testosterone. In fact, soy phytoestrogens do lower LH production in animals. This only happens after doses of soy phytoestrogens equal to 1.5 to 2 lb. of soybeans a day in man.

We think phytoestrogens may lessen the symptoms of menopause, but the estrogenic effect is much too weak to alter the growth and spread of prostate cancer.

Genistein

Genistein is the isoflavone found in highest concentration in soy. In the laboratory, this compound has a wide range of effects on human cancer cells, including prostate cancer.

Cancer needs more food and oxygen as it grows. The cancer forms new blood vessels to satisfy these needs (see Figure 4). When cancers can't form new blood vessels, their growth will stop. The process of forming new blood vessels is called angiogenesis and blocking this process is called antiangiogenesis. Genistein can prevent cancers from forming new blood vessels. This may play an important role in the ability of soy products to prevent the growth and spread of prostate cancer.

Prostate cancer cells are capable of committing suicide. This process of self-destruction can be triggered by a number of factors: when testosterone is removed following medical or surgical castration; when we treat prostate cancer with radiation or radioactive seeds; and when cancer chemotherapy drugs, such as Etoposide and Taxol, are administered. Genistein at high concentrations also causes cancer cells to enter this suicide program. The mechanism involved appears to be similar to that used by the chemotherapeutic drug, Etoposide. The use of Etoposide in the treatment of prostate cancer is covered in the January, 1997, issue of the ***Prostate Forum***.

The research on genistein is exciting, but there is one problem. Men on the standard Japanese diet have blood genistein levels that are only 5-10% of that needed to stop the growth or kill prostate cancer cells. There are only two possible explanations. First, genistein might be much more active in the human body than it is in the laboratory. Second, other compounds in soy might be more important than genistein.

Can Soy Make Your Cancer Shrink?

We know of only two reports of human prostate cancer responding to a soy product. The first study was conducted by

EcoNugenics, Inc using their fermented soy drink, Ecogen 851. A preliminary report of this study was published in the October, 1997, issue of the Cancer Communication Newsletter. At that point, a total of 14 patients were in the study. In clinical trials testing cancer chemotherapy, many investigators will call a PSA decline lasting longer than one or two months a "response". If you apply these criteria to the Ecogen 851 clinical trial, seven of the fourteen, or 50%, had a tumor response.

The scientific basis behind the Ecogen 851 product is interesting. In soybeans and most nonfermented soy products, the isoflavones, such as genistein, are bound to other molecules, commonly carbohydrates and sugars. Genistein and the other isoflavones must be freed from these molecules if they are to be absorbed. Normally this happens in the intestine. In the process of fermentation, genistein and the other isoflavones are freed from other molecules, speeding their absorption from the gut into the blood stream.

A range of fermented soy products is used in Japan and other parts of Asia. Genistein is generally more available in these products. In the case of Ecogen 851, the product is standardized for the amount of free genistein and other isoflavones and for freedom from contamination. Therefore, we can calculate the amount of genistein each patient received each day. All patients started with a daily dose of genistein and other isoflavones of approximately 26 mg, all in the free, unbound form. After some months, many patients' doses were reduced to 13 mg a day of genistein and other isoflavones.

This amount of genistein should yield blood and tissue levels that are still lower than those required in the laboratory to kill prostate cancer cells. There are two possible explanations for the greater-than-expected anticancer activity mentioned above. First, as we suggested earlier, genistein may be much more active in the human body than it is in the test tube. Second, in the case of fermented soy products, such as Ecogen 851, the process of fermentation may create new chemicals with much greater anticancer activity than those originally present in soy.

The Ecogen 851 clinical trial has not yet been reported in a standard medical journal. The importance of this is that when an

44

article reporting the results of a study are submitted to a standard medical journal, it receives an independent review by other scientists and physicians who look for defects in the study. It is standard practice to withhold final judgement until other investigators repeat a clinical trial to see if they obtain the same results.

A second paper reported the results obtained with a single patient. This patient took four capsules of a phytoestrogen preparation containing soy extract for one week before radical prostatectomy. At the time of surgery, a large proportion of the cancer cells appeared to be dying. One problem with this finding is that all prostate cancer specimens contain a mixture of healthy and dying cancer cells. It is really difficult to be confident that the phytoestrogen preparation increased the proportion of cancer cells that were dying.

Should You Use Soy?

We have no randomized controlled clinical trials showing that soy foods or soy isoflavones, such as genistein, have an impact on human prostate cancer. On the other hand, we do know that soy products are very safe. Additionally, they have many other health benefits, such as lessening your risk of heart disease. With these factors in mind, we think it is possible to make some recommendations.

If you do not now have prostate cancer and would like to prevent it, you may want to consider eating enough soy products to get 30 - 40 mg of genistein a day. Table 3 will help you in this process. If you find you like some of the soy products, eat as much as you like. It is safe and more may be better. If you find soy products unacceptable, you can take genistein capsules that are now widely available from many sources.

If you have prostate cancer, should you take soy products to slow the growth or spread of your cancer? The Japanese appear to get prostate cancer just as often as Americans do. The difference is that the cancer doesn't spread beyond the prostate gland as frequently in Japanese men. The implication of this observation is that the Japanese diet contains compounds that slow or even prevent the spread of prostate cancer from the prostate to distant sites such as the bone, liver or lung. The

Table 3. Genistein content in soy products.

Soy Product:	Genistein (mg in 4 oz):	Total Isoflavones (mg in 4 oz):
Textured Vegetable Protein	70-80	140-160
Soy Flour	80-90	115-130
Roasted Soy	80-100	160-180
Green Soy	70-90	140-160
Tofu	16-20	30-45
Tempeh	30-45	60-80
Miso Paste	20-30	40-50
Soy Cheese	2-20	7-30
Soy Hot Dog	8-10	15-20
Soy Milk	1-14	1.5-24
Soybean Flakes	50-160	65-270
Edamame (fresh green soybeans)	7-10	14-20

laboratory studies on genistein fit perfectly with this model: this isoflavone slows the growth of the cancer. The evidence does suggest that a diet high in soy foods might benefit someone with localized prostate cancer.

There are some patients in whom the cancer has already spread beyond the confines of the prostate gland to the bone, liver or lung. At this point, soy products would have to either kill or arrest the growth of prostate cancer for this approach to be of benefit for them. This is where the evidence is currently quite incomplete. The study by Kyle, et al., documents that genistein is capable of killing prostate cancer cells. The only problem is that the genistein content to be found in most soy foods is not enough. We would estimate that 500 to 1,000 mg of genistein would be required. If you consult Table 4, you will see that this would involve several pounds of soybeans a day or its equivalent. Perhaps concentrated genistein represent one solution to this problem. High doses of genistein can be accomplished with genistein capsules or drinks such as the Ecogen 851.

Soy in the USA

In the United States, we process soybeans in a manner that bears no relationship to the traditional Asian approach.

Soybeans are cracked, dehulled, flaked, and then soaked in hexane, an organic solvent obtained from petroleum refining, to remove the oil. The hexane is then drained off and evaporated, leaving the soy oil that you will find in your grocery store. The defatted flakes are then processed to produce a range of products including soy flour, grits and soy protein isolates. These defatted soy products are used as food additives such as a meat extender in everything from chili to hamburgers.

We think it is unsafe to assume that these soy products are comparable with those traditionally used in Asia, where their use is associated with a lower risk of cancer and heart disease. This is especially so because we can not fully account for the anticancer activity of soy. We are concerned that hexane extraction may lessen the potential anticancer activity of soy products. Unless the hexane is quite pure, chemical contaminants might be left behind when the hexane is evaporated. You may encounter the products resulting from this process, so we have listed them below:

Soy protein isolate is made from the hexane-extracted, fat-free, dehulled soybeans. The protein is extracted from the beans by dissolving the protein in water and letting the rest of the bean settle to the bottom. The protein-containing water is then treated with acid to clump the protein. The resulting material is more than 90% protein and is used in infant formulas and other products.

Soy protein concentrate is also made from hexane-extracted, fat-free, hulled soybeans. It is made by several methods, including washing the soy flour with acid, alcohol, or water after it has been cooked, leaving only 65% protein.

Soy flour or grits are made by milling the hexane-extracted, fat-free soy bean flakes. This material is only 45-50% protein.

Textured vegetable protein is made from soy protein isolates, concentrate, or the grits/flour just described. The soy product is subjected to heat, pressure, and is extruded into shapes that create a texture vaguely reminiscent of meat. Textured vegetable protein is often used as an extender for various ground meat products, such as hamburger or hot dogs.

These products could be very useful if you wish to incorporate soy products into standard American cuisine. We used these products many times in the past, but we no longer use them because of our concerns about the hexane-extraction process. In Chapter VIII we discuss traditional soy products.

References:

First, we list several references on prostate cancer in populations who eat soy products.

N. Breslow, et al. "Latent carcinoma of prostate at autopsy in seven areas" International Journal of Cancer 20: 680-688, 1977.

R. Yatani, et al. "Geographic pathology of latent prostatic cancer" International Journal of Cancer 29: 611- 616, 1982.

Next, we list references documenting the many benefits of consuming soy products.

Anderson, et al. "Meta-analysis of the effects of soy protein intake on serum lipids" New England Journal of Medicine 333: 276-282, 1995.

M. Brandi. "Flavonoids: biochemical effects and therapeutic applications" Bone Mineral 19: S3-S14, 1992

N. A. Breslau, et al. "Relationship of animal protein-rich diet to kidney stone formation and calcium metabolism" Journal of Clinical Endocrinology and Metabolism 66: 140-146, 1988.

C. Herman, et al. "Soybean phytoestrogen intake and cancer risk" Journal of Nutrition 125: 757S-770S, 1995.

M. Massina, et al. "Soy Intake and Cancer Risk: A Review of the In Vitro and In Vivo Data" Nutr. Cancer 21: 113-131, 1994.

Here, we list a reference on the economy of a soy-based agriculture.

R.P. Christiansen. "Efficacious use of food resources in the United States" USDA Technical Bulletin number 963, from the US Government Printing Office, Washington, DC.

Phytoestrogens

C. L. Hughes, Jr. "Effects of phytoestrogens on GnRH-induced luteinizing hormone secretion in ovariectomized rats" Reproductive Toxicology 1: 179-181, 1987.

Genistein

E. Kyle, et al. "Genistein-induced Apoptosis of Prostate Cancer Cells is Preceded by a Specific Decrease in Focal Adhesion Kinase Activity" Molecular Pharmacology 51: 193-200, 1997.

T. Fotsis, et al. "Genistein, a dietary-derived inhibitor of in vitro angiogenesis" Proceedings of the National Academy of Science USA 90: 2690-2694, 1993.

H. Adlercreutz, et al. "Plasma concentrations of phytoestrogens in Japanese men" Lancet 342: 1209-1210, 1993.

J. Markovits, et al. "Inhibitory effects of tyrosine kinase inhibitor genistein on mammalian DNA topoisomerase II" Cancer Research 49: 5111-5117, 1989.

T. Akiyama, et al. "Genistein, a specific inhibitor of tyrosine-specific protein kinases" Journal of Biologic Chemistry 262: 5592-5595, 1987.

S. Barnes, et al. "Soy isoflavones and cancer prevention: underlying biochemical and pharmacological issues" *Dietary Phytochemicals and Cancer Prevention.* R. Butrum, Ed. pp 87-100 Plenum Press, New York, NY.

J.R. Hebert, et al. "Nutritional and socioeconomic factors in relation to prostate cancer mortality: a cross-national study" Journal National Cancer Institute 90: 1637-1647, 1998.

M. Onozawa, et al. "Effects of soybean isoflavones on cell growth and apoptosis of the human prostate cancer cell line LNCaP" Japanese Journal of Clinical Oncology 28: 360-363, 1998.

J. Geller, et al. "Genistein inhibits the growth of human-patient BPH and prostate cancer in histoculture" Prostate 34: 75-79, 1998.

M. Pollard and P.H. Luckert. "Influence of isoflavones in soy protein isolates on development of induced prostate-related cancers in L-W rats" Nutrition Cancer 28: 41-45, 1997.

Wine

Red wine contains a wide range of natural compounds known to have anticancer activity. It contains epicatechins and catechins that account for the anticancer activity of green tea. It also contains quercetin, whose activity we have already discussed.

The French consume a diet high in meat and dairy fat, yet have a relatively low risk of heart disease. This has been associated with the consumption of red wine. The search for an explanation for this association led to the discovery of resveratrol, a powerful antioxidant able to slow the oxidation of cholesterol and lessen the rate at which cholesterol deposits in arteries. This compound is also a phytoestrogen. These same beneficial compounds may be found in grape juice, so you do not need to drink an alcoholic beverage.

To date, there is no evidence that consumption of red wine or grape juice alters the development or progression of prostate cancer. Consumption of one or two glasses of wine a night has documented health benefits in terms of a lower risk of heart disease, and may benefit your health in other ways, while giving you pleasure.

Reference:

G. J. Soles, et al. "Wine as a Biological Fluid – History, Production, and Role in Disease Prevention" Journal of Clinical Laboratory Analysis. 11: 287-313, 1997.

Chocolate

The chocolate that most Americans consume is made up of a number of ingredients. The most important component is cacao liquor. This contributes the brown color as well as much of the flavor and aroma. It is available in powdered form in most grocery stores. An example would be Hershey's Cocoa for baking.

Cacao liquor is then combined with cocoa butter to make baking chocolate that can be found in the baking section of the grocery store. Cocoa butter has nearly unique properties in that it is brittle at room temperature, yet melts at body temperature. In this form, the chocolate is quite bitter. However, if you were to add vanilla and sugar to this, you would have dark chocolate. If you also add milk, you would have milk chocolate that is so popular.

Chocolate is not usually characterized as a health food. However, the status of this food is now undergoing a reevaluation. One interesting property of chocolate is that it is very resistant to spoiling; unlike many other fats, chocolate does not easily oxidize or turn rancid. The components of cacao liquor are one reason for this. Polyphenol antioxidants make up 7 to 13% of the liquor. These include compounds we have already discussed, such as the epicatechins also found in green tea and Quercetin, which are known to have anticancer activity. Cocoa butter is composed of two fatty acids: stearic and palmitic acids. These are both saturated fat and are much more resistant to oxidation than the common unsaturated fats. This adds to the ability of chocolate to resist spoiling.

Stearic acid may also have a negative impact on prostate cancer cells. One of the largest studies of diet and prostate cancer examined the association between blood levels of fat and the risk of prostate cancer in close to 15,000 physicians. One of the interesting findings was that the physicians with the highest level of stearic acid had a 70% reduction in the risk of metastatic prostate cancer. Laboratory studies have confirmed that stearic acid does hinder the growth of prostate cancer cells. There have been no randomized clinical trials in which stearic acid or other components of chocolate have been tested for their impact on prostate cancer.

There remain some problems with chocolate. Milk chocolate contains butterfat and should be avoided. Sweet dark chocolate is available that contains no dairy products. Several studies suggest that chocolate may worsen diabetes mellitus. Additionally, chocolate is full of fat and therefore very high in calories. These are serious problems. Diabetes is often not diagnosed until serious chronic problems, such as kidney failure or loss of vision, develop. In fact, undiagnosed diabetes is one of the most common causes of impotence in men over 50! If you do not have a family history of diabetes and your physican assures you that you do not have and are not at risk of diabetes, it is likely that you can enjoy chocolate safely. It may even provide health benefits because of its polyphenol content.

There are some low-fat hot cocoa drinks commercially available. Most of these use low-or fat-free milk products. You can easily make a milk-free version that is also low in fat. The directions are in beverages in the recipe section.

References:

C. Sanbongi, et al. "Antioxidative Polyphenols Isolated from Theobroma Cacao" Journal of Agricultural & Food Chemistry 46: 454-457, 1998.

Osakabe N. Yamagishi M. Sanbongi C. Natsume M. Takizawa T. Osawa T. "The antioxidative substances in cacao liquor" Journal of Nutritional Science and Vitaminology 44: 313-321, 1998.

P. Gann, et al. "Prospective Study of Plasma Fatty Acids and Risk of Prostate Cancer" Journal of the National Cancer Institute 86: 281-286, 1994.

Grains

It is a common mistake to think of grains as solely a source of carbohydrate. Whole grains actually contain significant amounts of protein. The problem is that the protein available from grains is not high quality. By a fortuitous turn of events, the protein in grains nicely complements that found in most beans. This complementation of beans and grains allows vegans to satisfy all their needs for protein without resorting to animal products of any kind. There are many traditional recipes that made use of this complementation: succotash, pasta, and bean recipes from Italy, red beans and rice from New Orleans, or a Japanese dinner with rice and soy products.

The substitution of grains and beans for meat or full fat dairy products as protein sources also markedly reduces the total amount of fat in the diet. The kind of fat in the diet also changes: the vegan essentially eliminates one particularly troublesome fatty substance, arachidonic acid. Much of the remaining fat in the diet is likely to come from beans rather than grains. Here your choice can make a difference. Soybeans, for all of their benefits, have a high fat content compared with other beans. In contrast, Adzuki beans, widely used in Japan, have one of the lowest fat contents of any bean. If you are concerned with the fat content of soybeans, you can emphasize the use of low-fat beans such as the Adzuki. In that case, you may want to supply the missing soy isoflavones by using genistein capsules that are now widely available.

The bran of most commonly used grains is rich in a range of chemicals that can be beneficial to your health. This is one reason to use whole grains in your cooking. Table 4 contains a partial list of these compounds.

Table 4. Beneficial compounds in the bran of grains.

Phytic Acid
Lignans
Proanthocyanidins
Flavonoids
Ferulic Acid

Chapter 4:
Nutrition Becomes A Cuisine

MEAT-EATER, VEGETARIAN, OR VEGAN DIET?

These three diets differ mainly in the source of proteins. Most Americans use meat as their major source of protein. Vegetarians obtain their protein from dairy products and eggs as well as protein-rich plant products such as beans and grains. Vegans obtain proteins from plant products and rule out eggs and dairy products.

There is a link between the digestion of meat, dairy fat, and egg yolks and prostate cancer. Consequently, it would be prudent for you to limit your intake of meat, use only no-fat or low-fat dairy products, and use yolk-free egg products such as Eggbeaters. If you can manage a low-fat vegetarian lifestyle, you eliminate or reduce the fats most likely to fuel the development of prostate cancer.

In the Vegan diet, the major sources of protein are grains and beans. As we have discussed, grains and beans contain a range of compounds that may suppress the growth of prostate cancer. These compounds include isoflavones such as genistein and polyphenols. When you use grains and beans as your protein source, you reduce your intake of harmful fats such as those containing arachidonic acid while increasing your intake of the health-giving chemicals found in these plant products. This is why a Vegan lifestyle may well be the best diet for those concerned about prostate cancer. If you do adopt a strict Vegan diet, you should take supplements containing vitamin B12 and zinc as these are often not present in adequate amounts in plant products.

The major focus of this cookbook is to teach you how to prepare low-fat meals. The dishes that contain meat are limited to chicken and fish, because they are relatively low in the troublesome omega-6 fats. You will also encounter vegetarian and Vegan recipes.

Should you become a vegetarian or Vegan? There is no question that a low-fat Vegan diet will lead to the greatest decrease in dietary arachidonic acid and maximize your intake of the many health-giving natural chemicals found in plant products. There are several problems with this purist approach. First, many Americans balk at the idea of a Vegan diet. Second, the Vegan diet does involve developing an entirely new pattern of cooking and eating that takes time and energy to put into practice. Third, if you do any traveling, you will likely find it difficult to adhere to a Vegan diet. Fourth, you will need to be concerned about the zinc and vitamin B12 content of your diet. Fifth, there are no clinical trials that prove you need to go the extent of becoming a Vegan.

With all of these issues, we have adopted a flexible approach to diet. When it is possible, we eat a low-fat Vegan diet with occasional vegetarian meals. When we travel, we often find ourselves in a situation in which the best choices are low-fat fish or chicken dishes.

Cooking Style

Many patients tell us that they find it difficult to change their diet. The simplest solution is for you to adopt a low-fat version of the Mediterranean diet. Many Americans know and like Southern Italian cuisine and the ingredients are widely available. The staples of this diet are fruit, greens, pasta, beans, tomato sauce, garlic, olive oil, and red wine. In the June, 1998, issue of the Archives of Internal Medicine, de Lorgeril and colleagues reported the results of a randomized controlled trial that tested the value of the Mediterranean diet. Just over 600 patients admitted to the intensive care unit with their first heart attack were randomized to a control diet or the Mediterranean diet. After four years, the patients on the Mediterranean diet had 50% fewer heart attacks, about 60% fewer new cancers, and 50% fewer deaths. This diet is safe, tasty, easy to follow, and appears to have many health benefits. Judging from the number of Italian restaurants to be found in every city, Americans find the Mediterranean diet attractive. As an added benefit, Italian cuisine offers many vegetarian and Vegan alternatives such as spaghetti with marinara sauce and pasta with beans.

The cuisines of Japan and other Asian countries represent another alternative. These cuisines offer many examples of how to use soybeans and rice effectively, use neither eggs nor dairy products, and provide many Vegan dishes. Additionally, death rates from prostate cancer are low throughout Asia, a phenomenon that is easy to understand in view of the many chemicals in this diet with activity against prostate cancer. The proliferation of Asian restaurants attests to the popularity of Asian cuisine. The minute you switch from eating at a steak house to a sushi bar, you dramatically reduce the amount and change the nature of the fat in your diet.

In America, the cuisine of Mexico is often represented by dishes extremely high in fat, especially dairy fat, from the ubiquitous cheese. Regional Mexican cuisine contains many interesting vegetarian and Vegan meal plans. While not a low-fat option, we have been particularly taken with the Mexican use of baking chocolate in sauces. When used with discretion, it adds richness to the flavor without overwhelming the dish with the taste of chocolate. We hope you will try the low-fat version of chili incorporating cocoa powder or a square of bakers' chocolate. If you use cocoa powder, you get the polyphenols of chocolate without the fat.

In developing the recipes and meal plans in this book, we largely have depended on Mediterranean, Mexican, and Asian cuisines. We have made modifications to use widely available ingredients. Also, we have provided a range of simple recipes for everyday use, although there are some more complex dishes that you can use as the basis for a dinner party.

What To Do If You Travel?

It is quite a challenge to adhere to a low-fat, meatless diet while traveling. We have found several useful solutions.

Spaghetti with marinara (tomato) sauce is widely available. While some olive oil may be used in the preparation of the marinara sauce, olive oil appears to be one of the safer oils. Additionally, this dish is free of meat and provides plenty of lycopene. Other favorite Italian dishes are *pasta e fagoli* (pasta and beans) and vegetarian minestrone soup.

Sushi bars are a good choice. On a recent visit to a sushi bar, we had Miso soup (made from fermented soybeans), Edamame (young green soybeans briefly boiled in salted water), cucumber, and California sushi rolls. The latter contains a very small fragment of crabmeat. Our beverage was green tea.

There are an increasing number of other restaurants that also have a selection of vegetarian entries. Unfortunately, many of these are not low in fat. We make sure to question our waiter on the fat content of questionable menu entries and ask if fat can be eliminated. Salad bars can offer a useful alternative, although most of the salad dressings available have a very high fat content. One solution is to carry a small bottle of low-fat salad dressing with you. Or use individual foil-wrapped packages of fat-free Weight Watcher's Salad Dressings available in most large grocery stores and in some health food stores.

Reference:

M. de Lorgeril, et al. "Mediterranean Diet Pattern in a Radomized Trial: Prolonged Survival and Possible Reduced Cancer Rate" Archives of Internal Medicine 158: 1181-1187, 1998.

Hakim. "Mediterranean Diets and Cancer Prevention" Archives of Internal Medicine 158: 1169-1170, 1998.

Chapter 5:
Simple Rules to Live By

Eating a healthy diet is very easy if we abide by some very simple rules. We believe that the following guide may help you stay on the road to good health. Now we are sure that you have heard these suggestions many times. Be aware that they do work and you are what you eat.

Rule 1: Drink plenty of water, about 6-8 glasses each day. Add **lemons** for variety.

Rule 2: Eat plenty of foods containing fiber.

Rule 3: Eat **lots** of fresh fruits and vegetables every day.

Rule 4: Drink tea (especially green tea).

Rule 5: Distribute your calories among carbohydrates and proteins. Limit your intake of fats.

Rule 6: Eliminate all red meat from your diet.

Rule 7: Eliminate creamy, high-fat salad dressings and sauces.

Rule 8: Limit refined sugars.

Rule 9: Keep your fat intake below 20% of your daily calorie intake.

Rule 10: Take your vitamins and supplements each day.

Rule 11: Get plenty of exercise.

Rule 12: Get lots of fresh air and sunshine.

Rule 13: Read and listen to soothing music everyday. Learn how to relax.

Rule 14: Get enough sleep.

Chapter 6:
Do You Have to Change Your Whole Diet?

It is not necessary to become a total Vegan or vegetarian all at once. You can change your diet significantly by eliminating red meat. You will want to reduce your fat intake dramatically, and eat sweets and salt sparingly. You should include lots of vegetables, grains, cereals, and fruits in your daily diet. You may also eat moderate amounts of skinless chicken with as much fat as possible removed, and cooked with little or no oil. Fish is also a healthy choice, if eaten moderately. Salmon, which is high in omega-3 fatty acids, is especially healthful.

A Lacto-Vegetarian consumes grains, cereals, legumes, vegetables, fruits, and dairy products. A Lacto-Ovo-Vegetarian retains dairy products and eggs in their diet. To keep this type of diet healthy you should minimize your use of low- or no-fat dairy products. Egg whites can be consumed liberally, because they are the purest form of protein with no fat or cholesterol.

A Vegan eats grains, cereals, legumes, vegetables, and fruits. To be healthy and maintain a diet that includes all the vitamins and minerals your body needs you should learn to combine foods correctly. You should have a serving of brown rice with legumes (lentils, garbanzo beans, soybeans, navy beans, etc.). You can be creative and try other grains with legumes, sea vegetables, or traditional greens. Eating liberal amounts of cooked tomatoes, beets, and yellow vegetables, in addition to oranges, apricots, and pumpkin is helpful because they contain compounds called carotenoids (pigments in fruits and vegetables that give them their bright color) and they are excellent anti-oxidants. A Vegan or a vegetarian consumes three times as much folic acid as an omnivore, however the vegan diet does not provide vitamin B^{12}. It is wise to eat vitamin B^{12}-fortified cereals and foods. Soy products are a good source of high-quality protein, iron, vitamins, and minerals. You can incorporate soy products many different ways in your diet —

eating soybeans, tempeh, and tofu are a few examples. Tofu is very easy to cook or bake. It comes in extra firm, firm, soft, and silken forms. Extra firm and firm are excellent for grilling, marinating, or cutting large chunks to use in stir-fry meals. Soft tofu is great for sauces, gravies, dips, and pasta fillings. Silken tofu is wonderful in dessert recipes, milk shakes, and creamy soups. Although tofu is cholesterol-free and is low in saturated fat, it is high in total fat. This should not be of great concern because your diet would now be low in fat and soybeans are high in genistein.

If you use oil to cook, do not use canola oil. It is not recommended because it has a high concentration of linolenic acid. Olive oil is the only oil you will need because it is not saturated and is believed to be cancer neutral.

To summarize make sure you:

• eat plenty of fresh fruits and vegetables,

• consume fiber,

• omit as much fat from your diet as you can,

• totally eliminate red meat,

• limit any animal products to skinless chicken or fish,

• use as little oil as possible, or no oil at all,

• combine rice or grains with legumes and other fresh vegetables to insure proper nutrition.

Chapter 7:
What to Buy and Where to Buy It

EQUIPPING THE KITCHEN

We find a well-equipped kitchen makes our cooking chores much easier. Having the right tool for the right job saves time and frustration. Our equipment includes the following:

Blender

Crock-pot/slow cooker

Chopping knives

Colanders

Electric mixer

Food processor

Garlic presses

Glass canning jars (1/2 pints, pints, quarts, 1/2 gallons)

Ice cube trays, large and small

Ladles

Mortar and pestle

Mushroom brush

Nonstick cookware: skillets, pots, and pans

Nonstick utensils

Pepper mill

Pressure cooker

Ramekins

Rice/vegetable steamer

Ricer (to hand puree vegetables)

Spice grinder

Strainers

Vegetable peeler

Whisk

Wooden cutting boards

Wooden spoons

STOCKING THE KITCHEN WITH STAPLES

Our kitchens hold a variety of foods and staples used throughout this cookbook. We find that having these items on hand saves time and multiple marketing trips. You can trim expenses by buying in quantity.

Pasta

Lemon

Mushroom

Spinach

Tomato Basil

Whole Wheat

Shape

#9 (thin)

Acini di Pepe

Angel Hair

Ditalini

Farfalle

Fettuccini

Fusilli

Linguini

Orzo

Penne

Rigatoni

Ziti

Rice

Arborio

Basmati (white and brown)

Brown, short/long grain

Risotto

White Jasmine

Wild

Grains

Barley
Buckwheat
Bulgur
Groats
Job's Tears
Kamut
Kasha
Millet
Oats
Quinoa
Rye
Rye berries
Wheat berries

Peas

Green
Yellow

Beans

Aduke
Black
Butter beans
Cannelloni
Fava beans
Flagolette
Garbanzo beans
Great northern beans
Kidney
Lentils:
    Brown
    Green
    Red
    Yellow
Lima

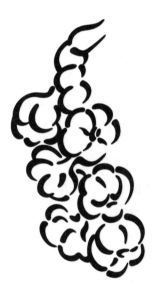

Navy

Pinto

Soy

Herbs and Spices

All Spice

Anise seed

Basil

Bay leaf

Black pepper

Caraway seed

Cardamom

Cayenne pepper

Celery seed

Chili powder

Cinnamon

Cloves

Coriander

Cumin, ground and seeds

Dill

Fennel

Fenugreek

Garam masala

Garlic

Ginger

Lemon rind

Marjoram

Mustard, ground and seeds

Nutmeg

Oregano

Parsley

Paprika (Hot Hungarian)

Poppy seed

Red pepper flakes

Rosemary

Saffron

Sage

Salt

Savory

Thyme

Turmeric

Wasabi powder

White

Vinegars

Balsamic (white/dark)

Cider

White

Wine

Flavored :

Dill

Garlic

Pepper

Oil (you only need one kind)

Olive

Extra Virgin: extracted from olives on the first pressing, cold-pressed without the use of heat or chemicals, having a pure fruity taste and a golden-to-pale-green hue, used as a flavoring and should not be heated.

Virgin: extracted from olives on the second pressing, cold-pressed also.

Olive oil: fits neither of the two descriptions above. Heat is usually used to extract the last bit of oil from the olives. This type is usually used for cooking over heat.

WHERE TO SHOP

In the United States we are fortunate to have large grocery markets that have organically-grown foods as well as those traditionally grown and raised. Many stores carry a good variety of fresh foods, vegetables, fruits, herbs, fish, and meats. Larger markets have beans, whole grains, and a large variety of rice and pasta. In many areas there are small ethnic grocery markets and natural and health food stores from which to supply your kitchen and provide many tasty meals. Choose stores that rotate their stock frequently for the freshest ingredients.

FROZEN FOODS

If you have difficulty obtaining fresh produce, frozen foods are an excellent alternative. They are picked at the height of their freshness, quickly blanched, and flash frozen.

You may wish to add small amounts of frozen vegetables to your recipes. For example, we frequently add a bit of corn to our dishes; the frozen corn is convenient.

STORING GRAINS AND BEANS

We use and recommend that you store grains and beans in tightly-lidded glass jars. Mason or bell jars in pints, quarts, and half gallons are very useful. We often save glass jars with good lids. We use glass jars because we can seal them tightly and odors are not picked up in the refrigerator. We use them both in our cupboards and in the freezer. Another advantage is that we can see exactly what and how much is in each jar. Labels attach and come off easily when we need to change them.

To use glass jars in the freezer, fill the jar within 1 1/2 inches from the top. Place the jar in the freezer on an angle. When the content is frozen, seal with the lid.

TASTEFUL AND HELPFUL TIPS

Many of us are busy either in our jobs or in retirement. Therefore, we offer some time-saving suggestions to make your cooking life easier.

EGGS

Most of the bacteria in eggs are between the shell and the inner membrane. Therefore, use an egg separator instead of the shells to separate the yolks from the whites.

GARLIC

In our recipes we use a lot of garlic in the Mediterranean tradition. We peel at least two whole heads of garlic at a time and store it in a tightly-lidded glass jar. It will keep in the refrigerator for up to two weeks. In our kitchens it is used in less than a week.

GINGER

Ginger brightens many dishes. Look for firm ginger, a sign of freshness. You may store it in the refrigerator in a paper bag or you can use our favorite method. Peel and cut gingerroot into two-inch lengths and store in a large glass jar filled with Taylor's sherry. This will keep in the refrigerator for several months.

OAT FLOUR

When a recipe calls for oat flour make it yourself. Use the food processor or blender to grind rolled oats into flour. It takes just a few minutes. Store the extra in tightly-lidded glass jars for future use.

OLIVE OIL

Olive oil can be expensive in small quantities. We prefer to buy olive oil in 1/2 gallon or gallon containers. These containers can be hard to handle. Therefore, we pour the oil into small, tightly-sealed glass bottles. It is best to store them away from light.

TOFU

Tofu takes on the flavor of anything in which you marinate or cook it. To express extra liquid from the tofu, place tofu between two plates and squeeze over the sink. If time permits, put a plate with a heavy object over the tofu in a shallow bowl. Let it sit for 30 minutes and then drain the excess liquid. To slice, set the tofu on a cutting board. Use a serrated knife to cut slices to the desired size.

WAFFLES

If you wish to keep waffles crisp do not stack them before serving. Use a single layer. Stacking them builds up moisture making them soggy.

EXTRAS

Rice and beans: When cooking rice, or beans we make a little extra to use in quick lunches or in the next days' meals. We store these in tightly-lidded containers in the refrigerator.

Vegetables: Instead of discarding the end pieces or vegetables near the end of their shelf life, put them in a pot of water and simmer to make stock. Remove the vegetables and throw them away. Pour cool stock into ice cube trays to freeze. When frozen, store the cubes in freezer-proof plastic bags. When you need a little bit of stock it will be handy.

Breadcrumbs: When you have stale bread of any description, don't throw it away. Get out your food processor, toss in the bread, and add oregano, basil, and powdered garlic. Pulse. Remove and store in tightly-lidded glass jars.

When we first started to cook and enjoy beans and grains we had a difficult time finding soaking and cooking charts. We have assembled a guide to make this easy for you.

GRAINS

Barley: Has a sweet, mellow taste and a chewy texture. A good source of fiber and minerals. It expands in cooking: 1 cup of dry will produce 3 to 4 cups cooked. Use 2 parts liquid to 1 part barley; bring to a boil, cover, reduce heat, and simmer for 40 minutes. Let stand, covered for 7 minutes.

Couscous: Staple of North Africa, made of durum wheat stripped of its bran and germ. A whole-wheat couscous is distributed by Neshamany Valley. It is brown rather than cream colored, because it is made from the whole grain. Bring 2 cups of liquid to a boil; whisk in 1 cup couscous; cook for 1 minute, whisking continuously. Cover pot, turn off heat, and let couscous absorb the liquid, about 5 to 10 minutes. Fluff with a fork.

Job's Tears: Looks like oversized pearl barley, is light brown with an indented stripe running down the middle. They are chewy and release starch in cooking, creating a slight stickiness. First, toast the grains in the oven on a baking sheet to assure that they will absorb water. Use 1 1/2 cups water to 1 cup of Job's Tears. Bring to a boil, reduce heat, and simmer for 1 hour. Let stand for 5 minutes.

Kasha: Most commonly available form of buckwheat. Use 2 parts liquid to 1 part Kasha. Bring to a boil, reduce heat, and watch very closely until liquid is all but absorbed. Immediately remove from heat. Let stand until the remaining liquid is absorbed.

Millet: A nutritional giant with a generous protein profile and large amounts of B vitamins, iron, potassium, magnesium, and phosphorus. It is easier to digest than many other grains. It stands up well to strong flavors. Use 2 to 2 1/2 parts liquid to 1 part millet. Bring to a boil and reduce heat after 5 minutes. Cover the pan and gently simmer for 20 minutes, then reduce heat to low, and let the grains finish cooking through for another 15 minutes. The grains should be fluffy when you remove the lid.

Quinoa (keenwa): Native to the Andes, about the size of sesame seeds. Has a more impressive protein profile than wheat and contains numerous amino acids. Use 2 parts liquid to 1 part quinoa, bring to a boil, reduce heat to low, cover, and simmer until all liquid is absorbed. Grains will appear fluffy.

RICE

Basmati Rice: Authentic basmati is imported from India or Pakistan. It has a nutty aroma and a chewy texture. Use 2 parts liquid to 1 part rice. Boil water and add rice. Stir and let boil again. Reduce heat, cover, and simmer for 25 minutes. Let stand for 5 minutes and then fluff with a fork.

Brown Rice: Nutritionally better because it has not been stripped of its hull, bran, and germ. It can be either short- or long-grained. Long grain is less chewy and fluffier than the short grain. Use 2 parts liquid to 1 part brown rice. Bring liquid to a boil and stir in rice. Reduce heat after a minute and simmer covered for 40 minutes. Do not remove lid for 10 minutes after removal from heat. The trapped steam will plump the grains.

Wild Rice: Not really a rice; but seeds of a native North American aquatic grass. Wild rice is high in protein and a good source of vitamin B. Use 3 to 4 parts liquid to 1 part wild rice. Bring liquid to a boil and stir in rice, reduce heat, cover tightly, and simmer for 45 minutes. Drain remaining liquid and let stand covered for 5 minutes. Fluff with a fork. One cup of wild rice yields about 4 cups cooked rice.

Wehani Rice: This mahogany-colored, whole-grain rice has a nutty flavor and is chewy in texture. Wehani was named by the Lundberg family rice growers of Richfield, Cal. Use 2 1/2 parts liquid to 1 part Wehani rice. Bring liquid and rice to a boil, reduce heat, cover, and simmer for 45 minutes. Do not remove the lid. Turn heat off and allow to stand covered for 15 minutes.

Wheat Berries: Cooked berries are always chewy, even when thoroughly cooked. Use 3 parts liquid to 1 part wheat berries. Bring to a boil, immediately reduce heat, and simmer for 1 1/2 hours. These instructions should also be used for kamut, spelt, rye, triticale, and oat groats.

BEANS

These guidelines are for SOAKED beans. Soaking reduces cooking time. If you do not soak the beans, they must be cooked 1/2 hour to 1 hour longer. Soaking the beans releases the gas-producing sugars into the soaking water, reducing the problem of flatulence. Soak most beans overnight, changing the water at least once. Replace water as needed, so beans are always covered with liquid. Small beans will be softened in approximately 4 hours. Make sure to discard the soaking water. In the following instructions reduce the liquid by 1 part if you have soaked the beans before cooking.

Bean cooking times vary so check about a 1/2 hour before the minimum time requirement. If not yet cooked, continue checking every 10 minutes or so.

Aduke: Also adzuki or auzki. Small, brownish-red beans with white stripes. These beans are a good source of vitamin B, calcium, and vitamin C, and are highly digestible. Use 3 parts liquid to 1 part beans. Bring to a boil, reduce heat and cover pan. Simmer for 1 1/2 to 2 hours.

Black Turtle Beans: Earthy and sweet tasting and make superb soup. Use 3 parts liquid to 1 part beans. Bring to a boil, reduce heat, cover, and simmer for 1 1/2 to 2 hours.

Black-eyed Peas: Probably introduced to the United States by slaves from Africa. They are relatively quick cooking requiring no pre-soaking. Use 3 parts water to 1 part beans. Bring to a boil, reduce heat, cover, and simmer for 1/2 hour.

Black Soybeans: Available at most health food stores. They are round and plump with a glossy skin and are an excellent source of high-quality protein. Use 3 parts water to 1 part beans. Bring to a boil, reduce heat, cover pot, and simmer for 2 to 3 hours.

Cannellini: White, oval-shaped beans. They are a favorite in Italy, the choice for *pasta e fagioli*. Use 3 parts water to 1 part beans. Bring to a boil, reduce heat, cover, and simmer for 1 to 1 1/2 hours.

Fava: Not readily available fresh in this country. Dried beans are oversized with a rust-brown colored skin. They have a tough skin that must be peeled. They are wonderful pureed. Use 3 parts water to 1 part beans. Bring to a boil, reduce heat, cover pot, and simmer for 1 1/2 to 2 hours.

Flageolets: A favorite in France. They are pale green in color, hard to find fresh, and are expensive. Use 3 parts water to 1 part beans. Bring to a boil, reduce heat, cover pot, and simmer for 1 to 1 1/2 hours. Serve with a drizzle of extra virgin olive oil.

Garbanzos (Chickpeas): Garbanzos are round and creamy in color, with a nutty flavor and a creamy texture. They are very easy to puree, making excellent sauces and dips. Use 3 parts water to 1 part beans. Bring to a boil, reduce heat, cover pot, and simmer for 1 1/2 to 2 hours.

Great Northern: These large white beans are grown in the midwestern part of the United States. They hold up well to cooking and have a very mild flavor. They can be used in heavily flavored dishes. Use 3 parts water to 1 part beans. Bring to a boil, reduce heat, cover pot, and simmer for 1 to 1 1/2 hours.

Kidney: Kidney beans come in a variety of colors. The dark red is the most widely used and is truly very popular in American cooking. This is the bean used in red beans and rice. Also, where would good old chili be without kidney beans? Use 3 parts water to 1 part beans. Bring to a boil, reduce heat, cover pot, and simmer for 1 1/2 to 2 hours.

Lentils: An ancient legume, a member of the pea family, lentils come in many varieties. There are green, red, pink, and yellow and, of course, lentils *le puys*. Lentils are high in protein and make a very good compliment to brown rice. Lentils do not require soaking. Use 3 parts water to 1 part washed and picked-over lentils. Bring to a boil, reduce heat, cover pot, and simmer for 3/4 hour. Be careful not to overcook, as lentils can become mushy.

Navy: Creamy, oval-shaped beans are the best for baked beans. Ideal for purees. Use 3 parts water to1 part beans. Bring to a boil, reduce heat, cover pot, and simmer for 1 1/2 to 2 hours.

Pinto: Southwestern beans, used for chili. Use 3 parts water to 1 part beans. Bring to a boil, reduce heat, cover pot, and simmer for 1 1/2 to 2 hours.

Scarlet Runner: Broad, flat, green pods with red seeds. You can eat the fresh whole bean or the dried inner seed. Use 3 parts water to 1 part beans. Bring to a boil, reduce heat, cover pot, and simmer for 1 1/2 to 2 hours.

Soybeans: Soybeans are very bland. They may be processed into tofu, tempeh, and soy sauce. We prefer black soybeans. Use 3 parts water to 1 part beans. Bring to a boil, reduce heat, cover pot, and simmer for 2 to 3 hours.

OUR LATEST DISCOVERY:

We always look for quicker and more convenient methods to prepare our foods. Recently we discovered that lentils and beans, as well as grains, cook splendidly in our rice steamer. We are so delighted with this method because the beans and lentils are fluffy and tender without being mushy. Most importantly this method requires only one step. You put them into the steamer

71

set the timer and forget them until they are done. Our rice steamer is the Black and Decker Flavor Scenter Steamer Deluxe HS 2776. It is plastic, not aluminum.

Chapter 8:
Traditional Soy Products

Soy products are a good source of protein and genistein. We list these products for your information and use in cooking and eating.

Roasted Soybeans: Soybeans can be roasted in the oven, heated in a skillet or even fried. The browned soybeans are then commonly salted. You can eat them just as you would peanuts. To minimize fat content, we recommend that you use dry roasted beans.

Green Soybeans: These are specific strains of soybeans that are best eaten as you would lima beans. Just steam or boil them in salted water while still in the pod. They can be eaten hot or chilled. They can be used in any dish that calls for lima beans. The Japanese call these beans Edamame. The fresh green soybeans are available in many Asian grocery stores. Out of season, we have found them in the frozen food sections. If you have a vegetable garden, they are easy to raise. Seeds are available from Park Seeds and Johnny's Select Seeds. Our current favorite is the Butterbean variety from Johnny's Select Seeds. Green soybeans can be grown in northern areas where limas do not do as well.

Black Soybeans: The usual soybeans found in health food stores are pale brown or beige. These are used in most of the recipes you might encounter. There are also black soybeans, which are well worth the search. Their skin is thinner, they cook more rapidly, and we find their flavor more appealing. They can readily be incorporated into many bean dishes.

Soy Flour: We prefer Japanese-style soy flour simply made from ground soybeans. This flour is used to make soy-milk and tofu. Our favorite is soy flour that has been toasted. In the European cooking tradition, browning flour is a standard step in making gravy. We find that this browned soy flour serves very well as a substitute. However, this flour is not fat-free: about 40% of the calories come from fat.

Soy Milk: This soy beverage is widely used in the United

States as a basis for nondairy infant formulas. Most health food stores and upscale grocery stores carry soy milk formulated for adults. For example, here in Charlottesville, Virginia, a town of less than 100,000, several brands of soy milk for adults are available. Soy milk comes plain or flavored with vanilla or chocolate. While we think these taste just fine, they do not at all remind us of cow's milk. If you are really attached to the taste of cow's milk, you can mix soy milk with skim milk. Another alternative that yields a very rich tasting drink is adding fat-free, dried instant milk to soy milk. Our favorite recipe is to put soy milk into a blender and add frozen strawberries, raspberries or blueberries until the mixture is too thick for the blender to stir. We add sugar and, at times, ginger to this mixture.

Tempeh: Tempeh is made by combining soybeans with grains such as barley or rice and then letting them ferment for a short period of time. The end result is a firm slab as thick as a hamburger. When cooked, it imparts a meaty flavor to a recipe. One way we use this is to fry it in a pan with a nonstick spray. When it has browned, we place it on a bun with mustard and onions. We also dice it into small cubes and add it to soups, stews or spaghetti sauce.

Tofu: Tofu was first used in China some time around 200 B.C. According to the Soyfoods Association of America the discovery of the process is lost to the ages. Ancient Chinese legend says that the first tofu was created by accident. A cook added *nigari,* a compound found in natural ocean water, to flavor pureed cooked soybeans and that produced the curd that we know today as tofu. Tofu is a dietary staple throughout Asia. It is made fresh daily in thousands of small tofu shops and sold in the street. Tofu acts like a sponge in recipes absorbing the flavor of anything that it is added to.

Tofu is made from soy milk by a process very similar to that used to make cheese from cow's milk. Calcium and other compounds are added to the soy milk to cause it to coagulate. The coagulated soy milk is then placed in wooden or stainless steel molds and excess water allowed to drain away.

Tofu is very bland in taste, but will take on the taste of whatever it is cooked with. It can be diced and mixed easily with soups or stews. We find it mixes well in the tomato sauce we use for spaghetti. Our favorite is to take one block of tofu, one cup of soy milk, and fresh or frozen blueberries, raspberries, blackberries or strawberries and mix them in a blender. Add 1 teaspoon of honey and a quarter of a teaspoon of ginger. If you wish, use skim milk instead of soy milk. The result is a milk shake that really tastes like a milk shake and not some substitute.

Tofu is rich in high-quality protein and is also an excellent source of B- vitamins and iron. When the curdling agent used to make tofu is a calcium salt, the tofu is a good source of calcium. Fifty percent of the calories in tofu come from fat. However, a four-ounce serving contains just 6 grams of fat. It is low in saturated fat and contains no cholesterol. Generally the softer the tofu, the lower the fat content. Tofu is also very low in sodium, making it a perfect food for people on sodium restricted diets. (See Table 5.)

Table 5. Nutrients in 4 ounces of tofu.

	Firm Tofu:	Soft Tofu:	Silken:
Calories	120	86	72
Protein (grams)	13	9	9.6
Carbohydrates (grams)	3	2	3.2
Fat (grams)	6	5	2.4
Saturated Fat (grams)	1	1	0
Cholesterol	0	0	0
Sodium (milligrams)	9	8	76
Fiber (grams)	1	0	0
Calcium (milligrams)	120	130	40
Iron (milligrams)	8	7	1
Percent of Calories from Protein	43	39	53
Percent of Calories from Carbohydrates	10	9	17
Percent of Calories from Fat	45	52	30

Source: Composition of Foods: Legumes and Legume Products. United States Department of Agriculture, Human Nutrition Information Service, Agriculture Handbook 8-16. Revised December, 1986.

Chapter 9:
Recipes for a Healthy Life:
So You Thought It Was Hard?!

Before we delve into our recipes, we offer a list of sample menus to guide you through the first week. These menus include a variety of the recipes contained in this book, **highlighted in bold**.

SAMPLE MENU

Day 1

Breakfast
Juice or fruit
Oatmeal
Green tea, coffee

Lunch
Mexicano Salad
Whole-wheat bread
Fruit
Green tea (hot or cold), skim milk

Dinner
Mediterranean Stew
Tossed salad with **Myers' Great Shakes Dressing**
Crusty whole grain bread
Peach Crisp
Green tea, coffee, skim milk, red wine

Day 2

Breakfast
Juice or fruit
Rosie's French Toast
Green tea, coffee

Lunch
Yellow and Green Split Pea Soup
Whole wheat bread
Fruit
Green tea (hot or cold), spring water with lemon, skim milk

Dinner
Tofu Cauliflower Stir-fry
Tossed salad with **Raspberry Vinaigrette**
Carrot Cake or fruit
Green tea, coffee, skim milk, red wine

Day 3
Breakfast
Juice or fruit
Omelet Delight
Green tea, coffee
Lunch
Mikey's Bean Salad
Whole-wheat bread
Fruit
Green tea (hot or cold), skim milk, water with lemon juice
Dinner
Jaiphur Chicken with Bulgar and Rice
    or **Kevan's Free Union Pie**
Tossed salad with **Apple Cider Vinaigrette**
Crusty whole-grain bread
Wease's Stuffed Baked Apples or fruit
Green tea, coffee, skim milk, red wine

Day 4
Breakfast
Juice or fruit
Snuffy's Blueberry Pancakes
Green tea, coffee, skim milk
Lunch
Pasta Primavera
Fruit
Green tea (hot or cold), skim milk, juice, water with lemon
Dinner
Red Bell Pepper Stuffed with Grains and Mint
Tossed salad with **Druhe's Special Dressing**
Greens
Rice Pudding or fruit
Green tea, coffee, skim milk, red wine

Day 5

Breakfast

Juice or fruit

Shredded wheat with skim milk or soy milk

Green tea, coffee

Lunch

Black Bean Soup

Crusty whole-wheat bread

Fruit

Green tea (hot or cold), skim milk, juice, water with lemon

Dinner

Ginny's Salmon or **Vegan Lasagne**

Oven-Browned Potatoes

Greens

Tossed salad with lemon wedges

Crusty whole-grain bread

Rosie's Mixed Fruit

Green tea, coffee, skim milk, red wine

Day 6

Breakfast

Juice or fruit

Oatmeal

Green tea, coffee

Lunch

Wheat Berry Salad

Crusty whole-wheat bread

Fruit

Green tea (hot or cold), skim milk, juice, water with lemon

Dinner

Chocolate Chili

Greens

Tossed Salad with **Ginger Lemon Soy Sauce**

Crusty whole-grain bread

Mixed Fruit over Angel Food Cake

Green tea, coffee, skim milk, red wine

Day 7

Breakfast

Juice or fruit

Diane's High Rise Waffles

Green tea, coffee

Lunch

Pumpkin Soup or **Sgarlat's Cucumber Soup**

Crusty rye bread

Fruit or a cookie

Green tea (hot or cold), skim milk, juice, water with lemon

Dinner

Rivanna River Clam Pasta
    or **Louise's Summer Casserole**

Tossed Salad with Savory Dressing

Crusty whole-grain bread

Cheese Cake al Tofu

Green tea, coffee, skim milk, red wine

Some handy foods to make in advance to add to various recipes.

ALL YOU NEED TO KNOW ABOUT STOCKS

We prefer to make our own stocks so that we can control the amount of fat and salt. We often make pure vegetable stock and occasionally a well-skimmed chicken stock. We do not use beef or pork.

Once the stock is made, it is convenient to freeze or store it in various-size containers. A great trick is to freeze a substantial amount in ice cube trays and transfer them to freezer bags or containers. A variety of sizes allows you to use whatever you need without waste.

Making the stock:
You can use a conventional pot, pressure cooker, or slow cooker/crockpot.

Vegetable Stock

SHOPPING LIST

Celery
Onions
Carrots
Green/yellow/red bell peppers
Leeks
Garlic
Basil
Pepper and salt, if you wish

PREPARATION

Pour a quart or more of cold water into a pot. Add diced and sliced vegetables. Slowly bring to a boil and immediately reduce to a simmer. Cook for 1 1/2 to 2 hours. Cool and blend in a blender, or food processor. You may strain all the vegetables leaving a clear broth.

Prep time: 15 minutes. Total time 2 1/4 hours.

Notes:

80

Chicken Stock

SHOPPING LIST
Chicken parts (skinned for the least amount of fat)
1 cup each of the vegetables
   Celery
   Onion
   Leeks
   Carrots
   Tomato
5 garlic cloves, crushed
1 tablespoon coriander
Pepper and salt to taste

PREPARATION
Pour a quart or more of cold water into your pot. Add chicken parts and bring to a boil. Add vegetables and spices; reduce to a simmer and cook for 1 1/2 to 2 hours. Place in a colander to remove the chicken and the vegetables. Cool the liquid in the refrigerator until the fat solidifies on the top. Take the stock from the refrigerator and carefully remove the fat. You may use the clear stock or add the vegetables and the chicken without the bones.

Prep time: 15 minutes. Total time: 2 1/4 hours.

Notes:

Miso

Miso can be purchased in oriental groceries, health food stores, and in some major chain stores. What is it? Miso is a fermented bean curd. Therefore, it is high in protein. You can add a tablespoon of miso directly to your food, or you can make a clear broth by mixing a tablespoon or two in a cup of boiling water. Some find miso too salty, so taste a little before you add it.

Notes:

Fish Stock

Fish (skinned for the least amount of fat, can use heads and tails, as well as the body)

SHOPPING LIST

1 cup each of the vegetables
   Celery
   Onion
   Leeks
   Carrots
Parsley
1 bay leaf
Pepper and salt to taste

PREPARATION

Pour a quart or more of cold water into your pot. Add the fish and bring to a boil. Add vegetables and spices, reduce to a simmer, and cook for 1 1/2 to 2 hours. To strain the stock from fish and vegetables, place in a colander. Cool the liquid in the refrigerator until the fat solidifies on the top. Take the stock from the refrigerator and carefully remove the fat. You may use the clear stock or add the vegetables and the fish without the bones.

Prep time: 15 minutes. Total time 2 1/4 hours.

Notes:

Chapter 10:

Beverages

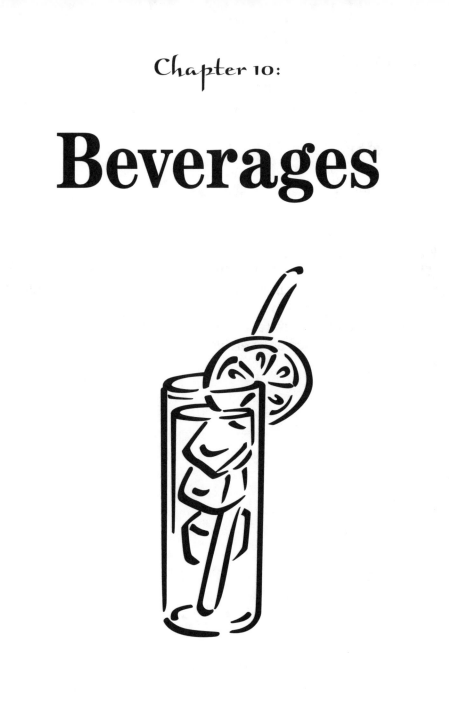

Green Tea

We have found that green tea can be rather bland; but if you add honey, ginger, and lemon it is quite tasty, if not downright delicious.

SHOPPING LIST
Green tea
Sugar or honey
Ginger
Lemon

PREPARATION
While boiling the water, put the tea and grated ginger in a tea ball. Place the tea ball in a teapot. Pour the boiling water into the teapot. Let the tea steep for 5 to 8 minutes. Remove the ball and add lemon and honey to taste. Serve the tea hot or cold. We often make large quantities and refrigerate it to cool.

Prep time: 15 minutes.

Notes:

Snuffy's Healthy Shake

If you crave a milkshake, but don't dare risk the fat, try this recipe to soothe your craving. You might never want a conventional milk shake again!

SHOPPING LIST
1/2 pound silken tofu
1 cup berries
1 teaspoon pure vanilla extract
1 cup skim milk

PREPARATION
In a blender, blend the milk and the tofu. Add the berries and the vanilla and continue to blend for 1 1/2 minutes. Pour into two chilled tall glasses and serve.

Prep time: 10 minutes. Serves 2.

Notes:

Low Fat Holiday Eggnog

This is a special and wonderful way to treat your holiday guests. It does have alcohol, but is virtually fat free.

SHOPPING LIST
8 ounces Eggbeaters
3 tablespoons sugar
1 quart skim milk
1 pint dark rum
4 ounces bourbon
1 pint nonfat frozen vanilla yogurt
1 teaspoon cinnamon
1 teaspoon nutmeg, freshly-grated

PREPARATION
In a food processor or blender mix eggbeaters and sugar. Gradually add half the milk, all of the bourbon and rum. Let stand for 10 minutes, then add the remaining milk, frozen yogurt, and cinnamon. Pour into a pretty punch bowl, sprinkle with nutmeg, and serve.

Prep time: 25 minutes. Serves 10 to 12.

Notes:

Hot Spiced Cider

This drink is wonderful after a morning or afternoon walk in chilly weather.

SHOPPING LIST

1 quart apple cider (homogenized and pasteurized)
2 to 3 cinnamon sticks
1 teaspoon ginger, freshly-grated
1/2 teaspoon nutmeg
1/2 teaspoon allspice

PREPARATION

Heat cider and add the spices, simmer for 10 minutes. Serve in festive mugs with a cinnamon stick.

Prep time: 15 Minutes. Serves 4.

Notes:

Hot Chocolate

Are you a chocoholic? This drink will make your day. It is delicious and is as smooth as the fatty variety. Note that the chocolate must be pure chocolate with no dairy fat.

SHOPPING LIST
1 quart skim milk
1/4 cup powdered unsweetened cocoa
1/3 cup water
1/4 cup sugar
Grated, dark, unsweetened chocolate

PREPARATION
Slowly heat water in a saucepan over lowest heat. Add sugar and cocoa. When mixture is well blended, slowly add skim milk. Serve in mugs with grated chocolate sprinkled on top.

Prep time: 15 minutes. Serves 4.

Notes:

Mulled Wine

This is one of our very favorite holiday or company drinks. It is festive enough for guests and is easy to prepare. All you need to add to this wonderful mulled wine are a few special friends, a chilly evening, and a blazing fire in the fireplace!!

SHOPPING LIST

2 cups water
1/2 cup sugar
4 cloves
6 sticks cinnamon
2 lemons, sliced thinly
1 orange, sliced thinly
1 bottle dry red wine
3 ounces brandy

PREPARATION

Bring water to a boil, reduce heat, and add sugar and the spices. Simmer for five minutes. Add the lemons and let stand for 10 minutes. Add the wine and brandy and heat gently; do not boil. Put the oranges into a punch bowl and add the mulled wine. Serve immediately.

Prep time: 30 minutes. Serves 12.

Notes:

Dressings
and
Sauces

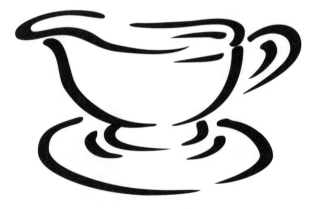

Druhe's Special Dressing

SHOPPING LIST
1 to 2 tablespoons mustard (Dijon)
4 to 5 garlic cloves, peeled and crushed
2 teaspoons extra virgin olive oil
1 teaspoon basil

PREPARATION
In a small bowl combine the ingredients. Mix thoroughly with a wooden spoon. Add mixture to Belgian endive or salad greens and toss to coat thoroughly. The recipe can be doubled or tripled for larger salads.

Prep time: 10 minutes.

Variations: Add 1 to 2 teaspoons honey or dried, sweetened cranberries, or slivered almonds.

Notes:

Savory Salad Dressing

SHOPPING LIST
1 teaspoon Dijon mustard
1/4 cup red wine vinegar
1/4 cup water
1/4 cup soy sauce
Dash tobasco (more if you dare)

PREPARATION
In a small bowl combine the ingredients and serve over baby field greens or your favorite salad greens.

Prep time: 5 minutes. Makes 2/3 cup.

Notes:

Myers' Great Shakes Italian Dressing

This recipe has evolved over the years to a point of perfection. It stores for a week unrefrigerated and, if placed in the refrigerator, for two weeks. Just remember to bring it to room temperature before serving.

SHOPPING LIST
1/2 cup extra virgin olive oil
1/2 cup balsamic vinegar
1/2 cup water
7 to 8 garlic cloves, peeled and crushed
1/2 teaspoon basil
1/2 teaspoon oregano
1/2 teaspoon freshly-ground coriander
1/2 teaspoon freshly-ground black pepper

PREPARATION
Combine ingredients in a bottle. Cork and shake thoroughly. Sprinkle over salad greens and mix to coat. Store in a cool place. Keeps for 1 to 2 weeks.

Prep time: 12 minutes. Yields 1 1/2 cups.

Notes:

Rice Vinegar Dressing

SHOPPING LIST
1/2 cup seasoned rice vinegar
1 teaspoon Dijon mustard
3 garlic cloves, peeled and crushed
1/2 teaspoon dill weed

PREPARATION
In a small bowl combine the ingredients and whisk for 1 minute. Add to salad greens or cooked vegetables. Store in a tightly-lidded glass jar in the refrigerator. Keeps for 2 to 3 weeks.

Prep time: 5 minutes. Yields 1/2 cup.

Notes:

Indian Curry Dressing

SHOPPING LIST
3 tablespoons seasoned rice vinegar
3 tablespoons frozen apple juice concentrate
2 teaspoons stone ground mustard
1 teaspoon lite soy sauce
1/2 teaspoon curry powder
1/4 teaspoon black pepper
1/4 teaspoon cumin

PREPARATION
Whisk the vinegar, apple juice concentrate, soy sauce, mustard, herbs, and spices in a small bowl. Add to salad greens. Excellent when served with spinach and apples.

Prep time: 5 minutes. Yields 1/3 cup.

Notes:

Dressings & Sauces

Sweet and Sour Salad Garnish

SHOPPING LIST
2 tablespoons lemon juice
1 teaspoon pure maple syrup
1/4 cup mint, finely-chopped
Pinch salt

PREPARATION
Mix ingredients in a small bowl. Toss with salad greens of your choice.

Prep time: 5 minutes.

Notes:

Apple Cider Vinaigrette

SHOPPING LIST
1/4 cup apple cider vinegar
2 tablespoons apple juice
2 tablespoons extra virgin olive oil
1/8 teaspoon black pepper
Pinch salt

PREPARATION
Mix ingredients together and let stand for 1 hour. Pour over greens of your choice.

Prep time: 5 minutes. Total time: 1 hour. Makes 1/2 cup.

Notes:

Ginger Lemon Soy Sauce

Ginger lemon soy sauce is a wonderful blend of flavors which will dress up any salad.

SHOPPING LIST
3 1/2 tablespoons soy sauce
3 tablespoons lemon juice
1 teaspoon ginger, freshly-grated

PREPARATION
Combine all ingredients and mix well. Toss with either fresh salad greens or pour over cooked vegetables of your choice.

Prep time: 5 minutes. Yields 1/2 cup.
Notes:

Lemon and Garlic Mint Sauce

This sauce is great on salad greens and even better on a blend of wild and brown rice. Dress it up with sprigs of parsley and a few slices of sweet red pepper.

SHOPPING LIST
1/3 cup lemon juice
1 1/2 tablespoons extra virgin olive oil
2 garlic cloves, crushed
1 tablespoon fresh mint, minced
1/8 teaspoon white pepper

PREPARATION
Combine and mix all ingredients well. Toss with either fresh salad greens or pour on cooked vegetables of your choice.

Prep time: 5 minutes. Yields 1/2 cup.

Notes:

Dressings & Sauces

Spicy Mango Condiment

Mangos are now widely available in North American super-markets and can provide an exotic fruity flavor, adding a zesty flavor to many dishes. Although many Americans have eaten mangos as a raw fruit, most do not know how good they can be when cooked. The following recipe makes a fruit sauce similar to a spicy Indian Chutney, which is delicious as a condiment, served on brown rice and lentil dishes where spiciness is appropriate. The sauce is sufficiently bold to stand up to dishes like barbecued or blackened fish and grilled poultry. It is also wonderful as a spicy spread on a slice of heavy sourdough bread. This recipe satisfies eight hungry people who are lovers of moderately spicy food.

SHOPPING LIST
4 ripe mangos
4 ounces Habanero peppers (+/-)
6 large garlic cloves (+/-)
1 tablespoon extra virgin olive oil
2 tablespoons balsamic vinegar
1/2 cup raw, brown sugar
1/2 cup raisins (variation)
2 tablespoons orange or lemon zest

PREPARATION
Garlic: Peel, crush, and lightly simmer in olive oil (do not brown). Cook 1 to 2 minutes in a microwave on lowest power.

Habaneros:
Wear latex gloves (important—trust us), wash and dry, remove vein and seed, then chop finely. Simmer peppers in vinegar; cook in a microwave on lowest power for 1 to 2 minutes.

Mangos:
Wash and dry, peel off skin and discard, then trim the flesh from the stone. Chop fruit flesh into chunks about 1/2 inch square. Stir in brown sugar. Combine ingredients (mixing well) and simmer until soft. Cook in a microwave about 10 minutes on a medium setting. Add optional raisins and/or zest before cooking.

Stir sauce again and refrigerate for an hour or more to allow flavors to mingle. Serve warm or cold. Mango sauce may be frozen for a reasonable time and is every bit as tasty when defrosted as when first served.

Prep time: 30 minutes. Total time: 1 1/2 hours. Serves 8.

Notes:

Raspberry Vinaigrette

Raspberry vinaigrette is one of the best reasons to have a salad. During the summer you can use fresh berries for an out-of-this-world dressing.

SHOPPING LIST

1 cup frozen raspberries, thawed
1/4 cup extra virgin olive oil
1/4 cup raspberry vinegar
1/2 cup water
1 tablespoon oregano
1 tablespoon basil
1 tablespoon parsley
1/8 teaspoon salt
1/2 teaspoon black pepper, freshly-ground
1/2 teaspoon sugar

PREPARATION

Put all ingredients in a blender and blend until smooth. Let stand for one hour and pour over greens of your choice. Store remainder in the refrigerator.

Prep time: 5 minutes. Total time: 1 hour. Makes 2 cups.

Notes:

Salads

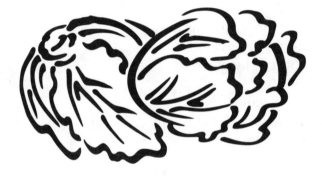

Mexicano Salad

Wonderful served for a special, but quick summer luncheon.

SHOPPING LIST

Beans

2 15-ounce cans black beans
1 15-ounce can garbanzo beans

Vegetables

1 green bell pepper, diced
1 red bell pepper, diced
3 plum tomatoes, diced
1 1/2 cups frozen and thawed corn
3/4 cup fresh cilantro, chopped
1 large red onion, finely-chopped

Dressing

3 tablespoons seasoned rice vinegar
3 tablespoons apple cider vinegar
1 lime, juiced
4 garlic cloves, minced
2 teaspoons cumin
1 teaspoon coriander
1/2 teaspoon black pepper, freshly-ground

PREPARATION

Drain, then rinse the beans in cold water. In a large bowl, combine the beans and the vegetables. In a small bowl, combine the dressing ingredients. Pour the dressing on the vegetables and toss gently. May be made in advance. Keeps well in the refrigerator.

Prep time: 20-25 minutes. Serves 8 to 10.

Notes:

Salads

Sara's Warm Cabbage

The combination of toasted walnuts, vinegars, and spices with the warm cabbage makes this a very special main dish salad! This is just the dish for a crisp fall day.

SHOPPING LIST

Main ingredients

1/4 cup walnuts, coarsely-chopped
2 tablespoons olive oil
1/4 cup balsamic vinegar
1 tablespoon apple cider vinegar
1 large red onion, thinly-sliced
2 garlic cloves, crushed
1 small red cabbage, thinly-sliced (5 to 6 cups)
1/4 teaspoon marjoram

Dressing

1 tart green apple, diced
1/4 cup raspberry vinegar
2 tablespoons parsley, chopped
1/4 teaspoon black pepper

PREPARATION

Toast the walnuts in a 350° F oven for 10 minutes. Heat the oil and the balsamic and apple cider vinegars in a large skillet. Add the onion and garlic and cook for three minutes on medium heat. Add the cabbage and marjoram.

Cook, turning gently, until the cabbage is wilted and the color changes from purple to bright pink. Remove from the heat; add the apple, additional vinegar, parsley, and pepper. Toss to mix.

Prep time: 30 minutes. Serves 6 people.

Notes:

Mikey's Bean Salad

Mikey first prepared this dish for us on a vacation to Smith Mountain Lake. Needless to say, this is an easy lunch dish for busy vacationers.

SHOPPING LIST

3 15-ounce cans of salt-free, red kidney beans
2 large red onions, diced
1/2 cup nonfat mayonnaise
1 teaspoon black pepper, coarsely-ground
1 teaspoon stone-ground mustard

PREPARATION

Drain the beans. In a small bowl, combine the mayonnaise, mustard, and pepper. Whisk together. In a large bowl, combine the beans and the onions. Add dressing and toss together.

Prep time: 15 minutes. Serves 6.

Notes:

Salads

Sgarlat's Cucumber Salad

This salad is great for a hot summer day and, on the other hand, is a tasty addition to a fancy meal.

SHOPPING LIST
3 large cucumbers, peeled if waxed
2 large plum tomatoes, diced
1 small red onion, chopped
1 teaspoon fresh basil
1/2 teaspoon dill weed
1/2 teaspoon black pepper
1 1/2 tablespoons fresh parsley, chopped
4 tablespoons thyme-flavored vinegar
Variation: 2 tablespoons nonfat yogurt or nonfat sour cream

PREPARATION
Slice the cucumbers and mix with diced tomatoes and onions. Toss the vegetables together in a salad bowl. Sprinkle the basil, dill, black pepper, and parsley over the top. Add vinegar and toss to mix. Chill for one hour.

Variations: Add nonfat yogurt or nonfat sour cream.

Prep time: 15 minutes. Total time: 1 1/4 hours. Serves 6.

Notes:

Rainbow Jubilee Salad

All the fresh vegetables served raw with this wonderful dressing are a colorful treat for the eye and the stomach!!

SHOPPING LIST

2 cups carrots, grated
1 cup red cabbage, shredded
1 cup zucchini, grated
1 cup turnip, grated
1 cup romaine, shredded
1 cup spinach, torn
1/2 cup radishes, sliced
1 small red onion, sliced and separated into rings
1 cup cherry tomatoes, cut in halves
Freshly-ground black pepper

PREPARATION

Combine all the vegetables except the onions and tomatoes. Toss with Myers' Great Shakes Italian Dressing. Garnish with onions, tomatoes, and pepper.

Variations: substitute dressing for one of your choice.

Prep time: 30 minutes. Serves 6 to 8.

Notes:

Salads

Summertime Vegetable Salad

This is a light, wonderful medley of fresh vegetables.

SHOPPING LIST

1 cup frozen corn
1 cup green beans, cut
1 cup carrots, sliced
1 cup yellow squash, sliced
1 cup red bell pepper, sliced
1 cup frozen peas
1/2 cup onion, thinly-sliced
1 cup oil-free salad dressing

PREPARATION:

Drop the corn, beans, carrots, and peas into boiling water. Cook for 3 minutes. Drain and plunge the vegetables into ice water. Drain and place in a large bowl. Add the remaining ingredients and toss well to mix. Chill for one hour.

Prep time: 30 minutes. Total time: 1 1/2 hours. Serves 6.

Notes:

Wheat Berry Salad

This salad is full of wonderful and spicy tastes. It keeps well in the refrigerator for 4 to 5 days.

SHOPPING LIST
3 cups cooked wheat berries
3 cups cooked brown rice
1 teaspoon orange peel, grated
3 tablespoons orange juice concentrate
2 tablespoons pineapple juice
1 tablespoon dry white wine
1 tablespoon white wine vinegar
1/2 cup vegetable stock
2 tablespoons extra virgin olive oil
1 naval orange, peeled
1 small head cauliflower, cut into florets
3/4 cup dried apricots, chopped
6 scallions, sliced thinly
1/4 cup chopped walnuts
1/4 cup raisins
1/4 cup dried cranberries
1 teaspoon dried oregano
1/8 teaspoon salt
1/8 teaspoon pepper
Parsley garnish

PREPARATION
Mix the wheat berries and rice in a large bowl. In a jar with a tight-fitting lid combine orange peel, orange juice, pineapple juice, wine, wine vinegar, stock, and oil. Shake to mix and pour over the wheat berry mixture. Put the orange into a food processorand pulse until it is in tiny chunks; stir into the grains. Steam the cauliflower over boiling water for 5 to 7 minutes. Mix the cauliflower, apricots, scallions, walnuts, cranberries, raisins, and oregano into the grains. Add salt and pepper, garnish with parsley, and serve.

Prep time: 2 1/4 hours. Serves 10.

Notes:

Salads

Pasta Primavera

Pasta primavera can be served as a salad or as a main course, either hot or cold. This is a colorful dish, which will enhance any table.

SHOPPING LIST
Main ingredients
2 pounds tri-colored pasta
1 cup carrots, diced
1 cup celery, diced
1 cup onion, diced
1 cup broccoli, finely-chopped
1 cup frozen peas, thawed
1 cup frozen corn, thawed
1 cup fresh fennel, finely-chopped
1/4 cup fresh parsley, minced
1/4 cup fresh basil, minced
1/4 cup coriander seeds
1/4 cup fennel seeds

Vinaigrette
3 tablespoons extra virgin olive oil
2 tablespoons balsamic vinegar or red wine vinegar
1 tablespoon oregano
4 garlic cloves, crushed

Garnish
Black olives, sliced
Vidalia onions, sliced

PREPARATION
Bring 3 quarts of water to a boil. Add the pasta and cook until *al dente*, then drain. In the meantime prepare the vegetables, except the corn and peas, by steaming in a rice steamer until *al dente*. Prepare the vinaigrette and let stand. Place the pasta in a very large bowl, stir in all of the vegetables, including the corn and peas, and the whole spices. Add the vinaigrette and toss to thoroughly mix. Decorate with sliced black olives and onion rings. This dish is an excellent one to serve for lunch or to complement any main dish. It keeps well for at least one week in the refrigerator.

Prep time: 1 hour. Serves 15.

Notes:

Mt. Fuji Noodle Salad

This recipe is in honor of a dear friend who will climb Mt. Fuji in the year 2004 to commemorate his climb in 1954.

SHOPPING LIST

Dressing
2 garlic cloves, minced
6 tablespoons rice vinegar
1/4 cup soy sauce
1 teaspoon Dijon mustard
2 teaspoons fresh ginger, grated
1/4 teaspoon red pepper flakes
1/4 cup light olive oil
salt and freshly-ground pepper to taste

Main Ingredients
1/2 pound Japanese (Udon) noodles or linguine broken in half
1 pound small, cooked shrimp
3 cucumbers, seeded and diced
6 scallions, white part only, sliced (reserve tops for garnish)
1 cup snow pea pods, sliced in thirds
6 leaves red cabbage
Garnish:
2 tablespoons sesame seeds, toasted
Scallion tops, sliced

PREPARATION

Combine all dressing ingredients, whisk in oil gradually until blended. Bring a large pot of water to a boil. Add noodles and cook until *al dente*. Rinse under cold water and drain. Put into a bowl. Add shrimp, cucumbers, scallions, and snow peas. Toss with noodles. Mix in dressing. Line a salad bowl with cabbage leaves. Fill with the noodle mixture. Sprinkle with sesame seeds and scallion tops and serve.

Prep time: 30 minutes. Serves 6 to 8.

Notes:

Salads

Chapter 11:

Breads

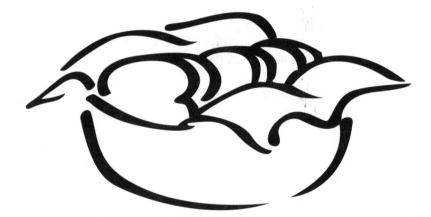

Sara's Garlicky Bread

This may also be prepared with Italian bread, but we prefer the baguette. This is a family and friends' favorite.

SHOPPING LIST

1 French baguette
6 to 8 large garlic cloves, crushed
2 tablespoons olive oil
3 Roma tomatoes, thinly sliced
1/4 cup Parmesan cheese or nonfat shredded mozzarella or
   provolone cheese
1/4 teaspoon basil
1/4 teaspoon oregano
freshly-ground pepper

PREPARATION

Cut baguette in half and slice both halves lengthwise. Drizzle with the olive oil. Spread the garlic evenly over halves. Place sliced tomatoes at intervals along the bread, sprinkle with basil, oregano, pepper, and cheese. Broil for 3 to 5 minutes to brown the bread lightly. Check constantly to avoid burning.

Prep time: 15 minutes. Serves 4.

Variation: Substitute nonfat provolone cheese or nonfat mozzarella.

Notes:

Breads

109

Minerva Jane's Whole Wheat Bread

This is a wonderful and delicious addition to any meal.

SHOPPING LIST

6 cups whole-wheat flour
1 cup white flour
1 cup bran flakes
2 cups oatmeal
1/2 cup wheat germ
1/2 teaspoon baking soda
1/4 cup caraway seeds
1/2 teaspoon sea salt
5 cups soy milk
Eggbeaters (2-egg equivalent)

PREPARATION

Heat the oven to 350° F. Mix the dry ingredients together. Mix the Eggbeaters with the soy milk and slowly add to the dry ingredients. Spoon into two bread pans sprayed with Olive Oil Pam and bake in the center of the oven for 1 1/4 to 1 1/4 hours. Cool on a wire rack.

Prep time: 1 3/4 hours. Serves 8.

Notes:

Sara's Low-Fat Bran Muffins

This is a great recipe for Bran muffins, not bland muffins. Add raisins or cranberries and you have a delightful dessert or a wonderful snack.

SHOPPING LIST

1 cup whole-wheat flour
1 teaspoon baking soda
1/4 teaspoon salt
1 1/2 cups bran
2 tablespoons apple butter
1 tablespoon brown sugar
2 tablespoons molasses
1/4 cup Eggbeaters
1 1/2 cups nonfat buttermilk or nonfat plain yogurt, thinned (by whisking) before measuring

Optional Additions (one or more)
1/2 cup raisins
1/2 cup chopped walnuts
1/2 cup dried cherries
1/2 cup dried cranberries

PREPARATION:

Sift the flour, baking soda, and salt together. Stir the bran into the dry mixture. Beat together the apple butter, sugar, and molasses; then add Eggbeaters and nonfat yogurt. Mix dry and wet ingredients, then add dried fruit and nuts. Fill paper muffin cups 1/2 full and bake in a preheated 375° F oven for 15 to 20 minutes.

Prep time: 15 minutes. Makes 12 muffins.

Notes:

Breads

Soups

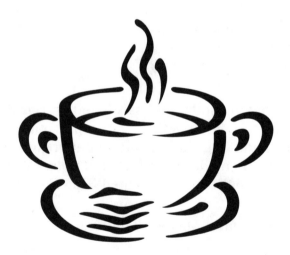

Provencal Soup

If you love soups, this will quickly become one of your favorites. This is great any time, especially when the herb garden has a bumper crop of fresh basil!

SHOPPING LIST

Main ingredients

1 1/2 tablespoons extra virgin olive oil

1/2 cup brown rice

1/2 pound fresh vegetables, such as green beans, trimmed and cut in half, zucchini, cut into thin sticks and/or peas, hulled

3 to 4 fresh carrots, peeled, and cut into chunks

4 new potatoes, scrubbed and sliced

1/2 cup small pasta of your choice

1/2 cup onions, diced

Pepper to taste

Dash tobacco

Pistou

4 to 5 garlic cloves, crushed

4 to 5 sprigs basil

1 teaspoon pine nuts (pignoli)

1/2 teaspoon extra virgin olive oil

1/2 lemon

PREPARATION

In a stockpot heat oil over low heat, add rice and onions, stirring until onions are softened. Add vegetables and stir until they are hot and coated. Do not let them scorch. Pour hot water over vegetables, enough to cover. Bring to a boil, cover, and cook on high heat for 10 minutes. Meanwhile, in a blender or food processor, blend together all the ingredients for the *pistou*. Reduce to a paste. You may need a trifle more oil; if you do, add 1/2 teaspoon. Set *pistou* aside. Drop pasta into the pot with the vegetables and cook until *al dente* about 4 to 5 minutes. Add pepper to taste. Now stir in the *pistou* and let stand for a few minutes. Serve in shallow bowls. Sprinkle with grated cheese, if you prefer.

Prep time: 1 hour. Serves 4.

Notes:

Minestrone Soup

This is the soup all Italians love. Now you can become a lover too.

SHOPPING LIST:

3 cups water

3 cups vegetable broth

2 cups tomatoes, chopped

1 cup carrots, sliced

1 cup celery, sliced

1 cup onion, chopped

3 tablespoons red wine

1 cup parsley, chopped

1 teaspoon dried oregano

2 cloves garlic, crushed

1/2 teaspoon salt or to taste

1 teaspoon pepper, coarsely-
   ground

2 cups zucchini, sliced

1 cup potatoes, diced and peeled

1 1/2 cups kidney beans, cooked

3 tablespoons small pasta

PREPARATION

Place water, broth, tomatoes, carrots, celery, onion, wine, oregano, garlic, salt, and pepper in an 8-quart pot. Bring to a boil and reduce heat and simmer uncovered for about 40 minutes. Add zucchini, beans, potatoes, parsley, and pasta. Cook for 20 minutes more or until potatoes are tender.

Prep time: 1 1/2 hours. Serves 8.

Variation: Use a 14-ounce can of whole tomatoes, undrained, instead of fresh tomatoes.

Notes:

Rose's Cucumber Soup

This is Rose's favorite soup for a festive occasion. It never fails to get rave reviews. It is easy to prepare and freezes well. If you plan to freeze it, eliminate the dill, the nonfat yogurt or sour cream, vinegar, and cream of wheat. Add these ingredients before you are ready to serve. This will preserve the fresh taste of the soup.

SHOPPING LIST

16 cucumbers 6-8" long
1 1/2 pounds leeks
8 shallots, chopped
1 large onion, chopped
8 garlic cloves, crushed
1 quart chicken stock or water
1/4 cup fresh dill or 2 tablespoons dried dill
Nonfat yogurt or sour cream
2 tablespoons vinegar
2 tablespoons cream of wheat

PREPARATION

Peel and chunk cucumbers, thoroughly wash and slice the leeks, peel and crush garlic and shallots. Place all in a large stockpot and add chicken stock or water. Cook until soft. Put through a food mill or food processor. Return to a large pot, add vinegar, bring to a boil, and then reduce to a simmer. Add the cream of wheat to thicken and season to taste. Add dill, yogurt, or sour cream before serving. May be served either cold or hot.

Prep time: 1 1/2 hours. Serves 8.

Notes:

Black Bean Soup

We first encountered this soup in a wonderful outdoor restaurant in Williamsburg, Va. We present our version of that flavorful soup. We learned the hard way to soak the beans overnight before cooking them and to cook them with a bay leaf.

SHOPPING LIST
1 cup dry black beans
6 cups water or vegetable stock
1 onion, chopped
2 teaspoons olive oil
2 stalks celery, diced
2 carrots, diced
1 large potato, diced
4 large garlic cloves, crushed
4 large shallots, crushed
1 teaspoon oregano
1/2 teaspoon black pepper
2 tablespoons lemon juice
1 bay leaf
Dash of liquid smoke
Salt to taste

PREPARATION
Rinse and soak beans in a quart and a half of water overnight. Pour off the water and put in a pot with 6 cups of water or stock and the bay leaf. Simmer until tender, approximately one and a-half-hours. Cook onion in olive oil until soft. Add diced celery, carrot, and potato. Stir constantly. Add the vegetables to the cooked beans, along with the garlic, shallots, oregano, and black pepper. Simmer one hour. Puree soup in a food mill, processor, or blender until smooth. Return soup to the pot and stir in lemon juice and salt. Heat and serve.

Prep time: 3 hours. Serves 8.

Notes:

Cabbage Garbanzo Soup

We love cabbage and garbanzo beans. Add the garlic and tomato, and we would say you have a perfect, hearty soup that stands alone as a meal.

SHOPPING LIST

2 teaspoons olive oil
1 large onion, chopped
3 garlic cloves, crushed
1 cup tomato, chopped
2 cups cabbage, chopped
1 large potato, diced
1/4 cup cilantro, chopped
4 cups water or vegetable stock
2 cups cooked garbanzo beans
1 teaspoon coriander
1/2 teaspoon cumin
1/2 teaspoon coarsely-ground black pepper
Salt to taste

PREPARATION

Sauté onion in olive oil in a large pot until soft. Add garlic, tomato, cabbage, potato, cilantro, beans, spices, and liquid. Simmer until vegetables are tender, approximately 20 minutes. Blend 3 cups of the soup until smooth. Return to the pot, stir to mix, add salt to taste.

Prep time: 45 minutes. Serves 6.

Notes:

Pumpkin Soup

This soup is not just for Halloween and Thanksgiving. It adds a touch "of the special" to any meal because of the wonderful combination of spices.

SHOPPING LIST
1 tablespoon olive oil
4 garlic cloves
1 large onion
1/8 teaspoon cayenne
1/4 teaspoon cinnamon
1/2 teaspoon cumin
1/2 teaspoon ginger
1/2 teaspoon mustard seeds
1/4 teaspoon salt
1/2 teaspoon turmeric
2 cups water or vegetable stock
1 15-ounce can pumpkin
1 to 2 tablespoons honey
2 cups skim milk
1 tablespoon lemon juice
1 tablespoon fresh cilantro, chopped as a garnish

PREPARATION
Heat oil in a large pot, add onion and garlic. Cook over medium heat until the onion is soft. Add mustard seed, turmeric, cayenne, cumin, ginger, cinnamon, and salt. Stir constantly. Add the water or vegetable stock, pumpkin, honey, and lemon juice. Simmer for 15 minutes. Stir in skim milk. Puree the soup in a food processor, blender, or food mill until smooth. Return the mixture to the pot and heat over medium heat until hot, but not boiling. Sprinkle with cilantro and serve.

Prep time: 1 hour. Serves 6.

Notes:

Mickey's Chicken Soup

Anytime we entered our Mother Mickey's house, the aroma of this soup greeted us at the door. Her chicken soup served as the pencillin for illness and the glue of family gatherings.

SHOPPING LIST

1 soup chicken, cut into parts and skinned
2 large onions, diced
3 celery stalks with leaves, diced
4 large carrots, diced
1 small tomato, diced
5 garlic cloves
2 teaspoons coriander
1/2 teaspoon black pepper
1/2 teaspoon basil
1/2 teaspoon oregano
1/2 teaspoon parsley
5 quarts water
1 cup rice or *acine de pepe*

PREPARATION

Wash the chicken and put into a large stockpot with the water and diced vegetables. Bring to a boil, reduce heat, and simmer for one hour. Remove the chicken, cool, debone, dice, and return it to the pot. Add spices, return to a boil, then add rice or *Acini di Pepe*. Boil for10 minutes, reduce heat, and serve.

Prep time: 2 1/2 hours. Serves 10.

Notes:

Potato Chili Soup

Potato chili soup is rich and smooth. It warms the soul on a cold wintry day, especially if you eat it in front of a fire after a brisk walk in the woods

SHOPPING LIST
2 large potatoes, diced
4 cups water
1 tablespoon olive oil
3 garlic cloves, crushed
1 large green bell pepper, diced
1 teaspoon cumin
1/2 teaspoon coriander
1 teaspoon basil
1/2 teaspoon black pepper
1 4-ounce can chiles, diced
2 cups skim milk
2 scallions, finely-chopped
Salt to taste

PREPARATION
Simmer diced potatoes in water in a covered pot until tender. Mash potatoes in the cooking water; leave some chunks. Set aside. Heat the oil in a large pot and cook the onion until soft. Add the garlic, bell pepper, and spices. Cook for 5 minutes. Add potatoes with the cooking liquid, the chiles, and milk. Stir and heat until hot. Garnish with chopped scallions and serve.

Prep time: 45 minutes. Serves 8.

Notes:

Green Silk Soup

Green silk aptly describes this delicious soup. We know it quickly will become one of your favorites. We love the name, too.

SHOPPING LIST
1 large onion
2 celery stalks, diced
2 potatoes, diced
2 shallots, diced
1 cup split peas
6 cups water or vegetable stock
2 medium zucchini, diced
1 stalk broccoli, chopped
4 cups spinach, chopped
1 teaspoon basil
1/2 teaspoon black pepper
1 tablespoon balsamic vinegar
Salt to taste

PREPARATION
Dice the vegetables. Put onion, celery, potatoes, and split peas in a large stockpot with the water or stock, and bring to a boil. Reduce the heat and simmer for one hour. Add zucchini, broccoli, spinach, spices, and simmer for 20 minutes. Puree the soup in a food processor, blender or food mill until smooth. Return the soup to the pot; add salt, balsamic vinegar, and heat. Serve.

Prep time: 1 3/4 hours. Serves 10.

Notes:

Barley and Lentil Soup

Barley and lentils go together like love and marriage. After you taste this soup, you will understand. Note that the spices in this concoction completely replace any fat.

SHOPPING LIST

1 cup lentils
1/2 cup medium barley
6 cups water or vegetable stock
1 medium onion
4 garlic cloves
2 celery stalks
3 carrots
1/2 teaspoon oregano
1/2 teaspoon cumin
1/4 teaspoon coriander
1/2 teaspoon black pepper
2 teaspoons tabasco sauce
1/4 teaspoon salt

PREPARATION

Dice vegetables. Combine all ingredients, with the exception of the salt, and bring to a boil. Reduce to a simmer and cover. Cook for one hour. Add salt and serve.

Prep time: 1 1/4 hours. Serve 8.

Notes:

Golden Beet and Potato Soup

Golden Beet and Potato Soup is a spring and fall favorite at the Myers' House. Why spring and fall? Beets are fresh at these times.

SHOPPING LIST

8 golden beets
4 large Yukon Gold potatoes
1 medium yellow onion
6 cups water or vegetable stock
1/2 teaspoon black pepper
2 garlic cloves
1 teaspoon olive oil
1/2 tablespoon dill

PREPARATION

Crush the garlic into the olive oil; let stand to marinate. Dice beets, potatoes, and onion. Put in a stockpot, add vegetable stock, and bring to a boil. Reduce heat and simmer until vegetables are tender. Add spices, crushed garlic, and oil. Garnish with dill and serve.

Prep time: 45 minutes. Serves 6.

Notes:

Fall Harvest Soup

There is something so inviting about the aroma of ginger, cinnamon, cumin, turmeric, and garlic simmering in a bit of olive oil. This recipe combines carrots and butternut squash with apple cider. It makes a great addition to your fall menu.

SHOPPING LIST
1 tablespoon olive oil
3 to 4 garlic cloves, crushed
2 shallots, diced
2 tablespoons ginger, shredded
1/8 teaspoon turmeric
1/8 teaspoon cumin
1/8 teaspoon cinnamon
8 carrots, sliced
3 cups butternut squash, cubed
5 cups water
1/2 cup apple cider
1/4 teaspoon cinnamon as garnish

PREPARATION
In a large stockpot heat oil and sauté garlic and shallots for 5 minutes until tender. Add shredded ginger and spices. Cook for three minutes. Stir in carrots and squash. Cook for five minutes. Add water and cider. Cover pot and simmer for 45 minutes. Stir occasionally. Remove from heat and puree in food processor, food mill, or blender until smooth. Return the soup to pot, reheat, garnish, and serve.

Prep time: 1 hour. Serves 6.

Notes:

Yellow and Green Split Pea Soup

If you are busy, this soup can be cooked in a crockpot on low for most of the day. It is wonderful soup to welcome you home from a hard day at work or play.

SHOPPING LIST

1 cup green split peas
1 cup yellow split peas
6 cups water, vegetable or chicken broth
1 large onion, chopped
1 large leek stalk, chopped
3 garlic cloves, crushed
2 shallots, chopped
2 large carrots, diced
2 celery stalks, diced
1 large potato, diced
1 teaspoon black pepper
1/4 teaspoon cloves, ground
1/4 teaspoon cumin, ground
1/8 teaspoon salt

PREPARATION

Rinse the peas and put into a large stockpot with all the ingredients, except the salt. Bring to a simmer, cover loosely, and cook until the peas are tender (approximately one hour). Or put the ingredients in a crockpot and cook on low. Blend one-half of the soup and return to the pot. Add salt to taste and serve.

Prep time: 1 1/4 hours. Serves 8.

Notes:

Rose's Butternut Squash Soup

Last year we planted our own butternut squash. This soup is the result of our experimentation with the home-grown variety. We have tried it with the squash from our local grocery stores and it tastes just as good.

SHOPPING LIST
4 pounds butternut squash
2 quarts stock
1 tablespoon cardamom
1 tablespoon brown sugar
1 tablespoon allspice
1 tablespoon cinnamon
1 tablespoon nutmeg
2 tablespoons low-fat peanut butter

PREPARATION
Wash and cut the squash into sections. Remove seeds. Put in a large pot, cover with water, and cook over medium heat until soft. Drain, reserving 1 quart of the cooking water. Run cold water over the squash and drain. Scoop the squash from the skins and blend in a food processor until smooth. Add the squash to a large pot with 2 quarts of stock. Stir, mixing the liquid and squash. Add some of the cooking water to thin. Add the spices, sugar, and cook over low heat simmering for 1/2 hour. Add the peanut butter and stir until completely mixed. Cook 15 minutes longer.

Prep time: 45 minutes. Total time: 2 hours. Serves 8.

Notes:

Mushroom Potato and Barley Soup Supreme

This soup is rich and savory. It is the perfect beginning to an elegant dinner or is wonderful as a meal by itself with crusty bread, a simple salad, and a glass of cabernet sauvignon.

SHOPPING LIST

3 large golden potatoes, diced
1 cup dried mushrooms (shiitake, maitake, oyster)
1/2 cup barley
1/4 lb red Swiss chard, chopped
4 quarts water
1 teaspoon hot Hungarian paprika
1/2 teaspoon hot curry powder
1/2 teaspoon ground coriander
1/2 teaspoon ginger
1/2 teaspoon turmeric
1/2 teaspoon marjoram (fresh or dried)
1 teaspoon of fresh rosemary
1/2 teaspoon thyme
1/2 teaspoon dill
1/2 teaspoon fresh basil
1/5 cup soy sauce
3 to 4 garlic cloves, crushed
Salt and pepper to taste

PREPARATION

In a stockpot bring the water, mushrooms, and potatoes to a boil. Add the barley. Reduce heat to simmer, add the spices, and cook for 45 minutes. Five minutes before serving add the Swiss chard and cook until *al dente*. Serve.

Prep time: 1 hour. Serves 4 to 6.

Notes:

Buck Mountain Mushroom Soup

This is a very simple soup and simply delicious when made with very fresh mushrooms.

SHOPPING LIST

2 cups fresh maitake mushrooms
1 onion, chopped
4-5 garlic cloves, crushed
2 tablespoons lemon juice
4 cups water, chicken, or vegetable broth

PREPARATION

In a blender, blend the mushrooms with a small portion of the broth; then add to the remaining broth in a stockpot. Add the onions, lemon juice, and garlic. Bring to a boil, then reduce heat to a simmer, and cook for one-half hour. Add salt and pepper to taste.

Prep time: 45 minutes. Serves 4.

Notes:

Chapter 12:

Main Courses

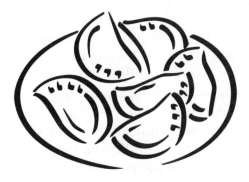

Tofu Cauliflower Stir-fry

This is a great way to try tofu if you must be convinced that you can make it taste good!! The marinade is very flavorful. You can add more garlic or more ginger if you are so inclined.

SHOPPING LIST

Marinade

2 tablespoons tamari soy sauce
1 tablespoon malt vinegar
2 teaspoons apple cider vinegar
3 garlic cloves, peeled and crushed
1 tablespoon ginger, grated
1 tablespoon olive oil

Stir-fry

1 tablespoon olive oil
1 large onion, chopped
2 large garlic cloves, chopped
1 pound firm tofu, drained, cut into 1" cubes
3 cups kale leaves, chopped and tightly-packed
1 1/2 tablespoons mild curry powder
1/4 teaspoon ground cinnamon
1/2 teaspoon saffron
1 1/2 cups vegetable stock or miso
1 large head of cauliflower, cut into florets
1 large red bell pepper, seeded and diced
1 teaspoon tamari soy sauce
1/4 cup parsley or cilantro, minced and tightly-packed

PREPARATION

Marinate tofu for 25 minutes in the refrigerator before cooking. In a large skillet or wok heat the oil and add onion, garlic, and tofu. Sauté until the tofu is brown. Stir in the kale and sprinkle on the cinnamon, saffron, and curry powder. Add 1/4 cup of the broth, cover, and cook over medium heat for 2 minutes. Then add the cauliflower, red pepper, and sprinkle with tamari. Add 1/2 cup broth, cover and continue to cook, stirring every minute or so until the kale is tender and the cauliflower is *al dente*, about 5 minutes. Add more broth as needed to prevent burning. Stir in the parsley or cilantro. Add more soy sauce if needed. May be served over rice, bulgur, or couscous.

Prep time: 45 minutes. Serves 6.

Variations:

1. Substitute pureed tomatoes for all or a part of the broth.

2. Add a small, red hot pepper or a large pinch of crushed red pepper flakes.

Notes:

Rivanna River Clam Pasta

We began with a favorite Italian recipe for clam pasta and added wine and bourbon. The olive oil can be reduced or eliminated. If eliminated, cook onion and garlic in a nonstick pan with a bit of the stock. The clam stock, chicken stock, and wine make a rich flavorful broth; and the bourbon adds a dash of excitement.

SHOPPING LIST
3 dozen cherry-stone clams, washed thoroughly
1 tablespoon oatmeal
1 1/2 tablespoons olive oil
1 medium onion, finely-chopped
3 large garlic cloves, crushed
2 cups chicken stock
1/4 cup dry white wine
1 pound whole-wheat pasta
1 teaspoon bourbon
1/2 teaspoon ground or flaked red pepper

PREPARATION
To clean the clams; place them in a large bowl. Add cold water to cover, and stir in the oatmeal. Let stand 15 minutes. Rinse several times under cold running water and drain.

Heat the oil in a large saucepan over medium-low heat, add the onion, and cook for 1 minute. Add the garlic and cook 4 minutes longer. Add the clams, stock, and wine and heat to boiling. Reduce the heat and cook covered until the clams open. Remove the clams from the broth and place in a bowl. Remove the clam meat from the shells. Catch all the juices. Add the juices to the broth and boil until reduced by about one third. Coarsely chop the clams. In the meantime cook the pasta until *al dente* or tender. Drain. Combine the pasta, clams, and broth and toss until warmed through. Add the pepper and the bourbon.

Prep time: 45 minutes. Total time 1 hour. Serves 4.

Notes:

Jaiphur Chicken with Bulgur and Rice

For a tasty meal, serve with salad and a green vegetable. This dish is a great introduction to bulgur if you have not experienced it before. The combination of ingredients and the method of cooking bring out the wonderful nutty flavor of the bulgur.

SHOPPING LIST

1/2 cup bulgur
1/2 cup long grain brown basmati rice
1 tablespoon olive oil
3 pounds chicken, skinned and deboned
1 large onion, chopped
4 large garlic cloves, crushed
1/2 teaspoon turmeric
1/4 teaspoon ground cumin
2 teaspoons fennel seeds
1/2 teaspoon cayenne pepper
1/2 teaspoon black pepper, freshly-ground
1/2 teaspoon paprika
1/2 cup water
For garnish, fresh parsley, chopped

PREPARATION

Cook the bulgur in a large pot of water for 10 minutes. Add the rice and return to a boil; cook for 15 minutes longer. Drain. Place the colander over 2 inches of boiling water in another pot. Make sure the colander is above the water. Cover the bulgur and rice mixture with a single layer of paper towels. Steam for 15 minutes. In the meantime heat the oil in a large, heavy skillet over medium heat. Sauté the chicken a few pieces at a time, until well browned. Transfer all of the chicken to a plate. Blend all of the spices and the garlic until smooth. In the skillet add the onion and cook over medium-low heat, scraping the bottom and sides of the pan. Stir in the blended spice and garlic mixture. Cook for two minutes longer. Stir in the water and return the chicken to the pan. Bring to a boil and then reduce to a simmer. Cover. Baste occasionally until the chicken is cooked. Takes about 40 minutes. To serve, fluff the bulgur/rice mixture and arrange around the edges of a serving platter. Spoon the chicken mixture into the center. Garnish with parsley.

Prep time: 1 1/2 hours. Serves 4.

Notes:

Red Bell Pepper Stuffed with Grains and Mint

This is a dish Sara serves at Thanksgiving as an alternative to turkey. This meal is made very festive with the red bell peppers, and the flavor is delicate and sweet.

SHOPPING LIST

1 cup millet
1 3/4 cups vegetable broth
1 medium red onion, finely-chopped
2 celery stalks, finely-chopped
2 garlic cloves, crushed
1 cup frozen corn, thawed
1 tablespoon fresh mint, chopped
2 teaspoons lemon zest
1 1/2 teaspoons fresh oregano, minced or 1/2 teaspoon dried
1 teaspoon dried, ground black pepper
4 medium red bell peppers, tops removed, seeded and ribbed
1 1/2 tablespoons extra virgin olive oil
2 tablespoons fresh lemon juice

PREPARATION

Wash millet by placing it in a fine mesh strainer and rinse it under cool water. To cook, use 2 parts broth to 1 part millet. Bring to a boil, and reduce heat after 3 minutes. Cover and simmer gently for 20 minutes on low heat. Turn the burner off and let the millet steam for 15 minutes. Let cool for 15 to 20 minutes. Fluff with a fork. Add onion, celery, garlic, corn, mint, lemon zest, and oregano. Blend and season to taste with ground pepper. Cut a very thin slice off the bottom of each red pepper, taking care not to pierce. Stuff each pepper with millet mixture. Brush or drizzle top of each pepper with a bit of the olive oil. Place peppers in a rectangular baking pan, just large enough to hold them. Add water to the baking dish, up to 1 inch. Place in the center rack of the oven. Bake in preheated oven at 375° F for 60 minutes. In a small bowl, whisk together the remaining oil and lemon juice. Spoon a bit of this dressing into each pepper before serving.

Prep time: 1 hour and 20 minutes. Serves 4.

Notes:

Quinoa Classic with Potato and Corn

This is a wonderful, rich, and savory dish. We love it the most after a day hiking in the woods in the late fall. However, we think you might like it anytime

SHOPPING LIST

1 large onion, chopped coarsely
4 garlic cloves, crushed
1 tablespoon olive oil
2 cups potatoes, diced
2 cups vegetable stock
1 1/2 cups uncooked quinoa, rinsed
1 3/4 cups frozen corn
1 teaspoon dried oregano
1 teaspoon tarragon
1 teaspoon red pepper flakes
Freshly-ground black pepper

PREPARATION

Sauté onion and garlic in oil in a large skillet, over medium heat until onion is soft. Add potatoes and sauté for an additional 2 minutes. Pour in the vegetable stock, quinoa, corn, oregano, tarragon, and red pepper flakes. Bring to a boil, then lower heat and cover the skillet. Simmer 20 minutes or until all liquid has been absorbed. Add pepper to taste and serve.

Prep time: 1/2 hour. Serves 6.

Notes:

Italian Riviera Garbanzo

Not only is this a very tasty dish, but it is beautiful as well. We love the flavor of garbanzos especially when combined with garlic, olive oil, and roma tomatoes. Try this with your favorite grains or with pasta. You can use canned garbanzos if you are in a hurry, but cooking the beans yourself certainly lowers the sodium content.

SHOPPING LIST

4 garlic cloves, crushed
1 tablespoon olive oil
3 cups cooked garbanzos
1 10-ounce package frozen spinach, defrosted
1 large red onion, chopped
1 28-ounce can crushed tomatoes, (no salt/ or low sodium)
1 cup Roma tomatoes, chopped
1 tablespoon crushed red pepper
1 shallot, chopped
1 tablespoon oregano
2 lemons, juiced
Freshly-ground black pepper

PREPARATION

Sauté the onion and garlic in olive oil in a large saucepan over medium heat until onions are soft. Add the garbanzos, spinach, tomatoes, pepper flakes, shallot and oregano. Cover and simmer for 30 minutes. Add lemon juice and ground black pepper.

Prep time: 45 minutes. Serves 8.

Notes:

Chocolate Chili

This has become one our favorite recipes. It is delicious and rich. Just right for an evening by the fireplace. Do you think it is the chocolate?

SHOPPING LIST
1 large onion, coarsely-chopped
1 large green bell pepper, seeded and chopped
1 tablespoon olive oil
1 tablespoon whole mustard seed
1 square Ghiradelli dark chocolate (no milk fat)
1 teaspoon ground cinnamon
2 tablespoons chili powder
1 teaspoon whole cumin seeds
1 16-ounce can crushed tomatoes
2 16-ounce cans pinto or red beans, with liquid
1 6-ounce can tomato paste

PREPARATION
In a large saucepan sauté the onion and green pepper in the olive oil over medium heat until onions are lightly browned. Add mustard seed and cook, stirring for 2 minutes. Add chili powder, cumin seed, square of chocolate, cinnamon, tomatoes, beans with liquid, and tomato paste. Simmer gently, uncovered, for about 35 minutes, stirring frequently, until the chili is thick. Serve with crusty bread, a green salad, and a glass of cabernet.

Prep. Time: 1 1/4 hours. Serves 6.

Notes:

Hearty Lentil, Barley, Bean, and Vegetable Stew

This stew is a good winter meal and is very satisfying served with a French baguette and a crisp green salad.

SHOPPING LIST

1 1/2 tablespoons olive oil
4 carrots, diced to 1/4"
2 leeks, diced to 1/4"
2 ribs of celery, diced to 1/4"
1 large onion, chopped coarsely
2 medium zucchini, cut into 1/4" pieces
2 to 3 garlic cloves, crushed
1 tablespoon fresh thyme leaves: or
   1 teaspoon dried thyme
1 cup dried lentils, rinsed and picked-over
1/2 cup pearl barley, rinsed
1/2 cup cooked white beans
7 cups concentrated vegetable broth
2 cups tomatoes, seeded and chopped
1 cup fresh basil, torn
1/2 cup parsley, coarsely-chopped
Pepper to taste

PREPARATION

Place oil in a large, heavy pot and add carrots, leeks, celery, zucchini, onion and garlic. Cook over low heat, stirring until the vegetables are wilted, about 15 minutes. Add lentils, barley, and 6 cups of the broth. Bring to a boil, reduce to medium heat, and simmer for 30 minutes. Add tomatoes, basil, and cooked white beans. Season with ground pepper and cook 10 minutes more. Stir in parsley. Add in the last cup of vegetable broth and stir gently.

Be careful not to overcook.

Prep time: 1 1/4 hours. Serves 6.

Notes:

Stacy's Dead of Winter Brown Rice Chili

This is another wonderful dish made with beans. It has a "salt of the earth" flavor.

SHOPPING LIST
1 tablespoon olive oil
1 large yellow onion, chopped
1 green bell pepper, chopped and seeded
2 ribs of celery, diced
4 to 5 garlic cloves, crushed
1 28 ounce can stewed tomatoes with juice
1 15-ounce can red kidney beans, rinsed and drained
1 15-ounce can pinto beans, rinsed and drained
1 15-ounce can chickpeas, rinsed and drained
1 cup frozen corn
3 Jalapeno peppers, chopped and seeded
1 small can chili peppers
1 cup uncooked brown rice
2 tablespoons chili powder
1 tablespoon dried oregano
1 1/2 teaspoons ground cumin
1/2 tablespoon black pepper

PREPARATION
Heat oil in a large saucepan over medium-high heat. Add onion, bell pepper, celery, and garlic. Cook, stirring for 7 minutes. Stir in tomatoes, all the beans, corn, water, peppers, rice, and seasonings. Bring to a simmer, cover, and cook over medium-low heat until rice is tender, about 40 minutes. Stir occasionally near the end of cooking. Remove chili from heat. Let stand for 15 minutes.

Prep time: 1 1/2 hours. Serves 8.

Notes:

Main Courses

Mediterranean Stew

Once you taste this stew you will think you were born Italian, Greek, or French. It will quickly become one of your staple recipes.

SHOPPING LIST
1 large eggplant, thinly-sliced
1 pound tiny new potatoes
1 cup vegetable broth
2 tablespoons balsamic vinegar
1 large onion, chopped
2 shallots, chopped
2 tablespoons grated ginger
1/4 cup fresh basil, minced
2 teaspoons ground cumin
2 teaspoons ground coriander
2 teaspoons cinnamon
1/2 teaspoon saffron
2 red bell peppers, roasted and thinly-sliced
1 green bell pepper, roasted and thinly-sliced
1 yellow bell pepper roasted and thinly-sliced
3 cups cooked chickpeas (garbanzo beans)
1 1/2 cups fresh roma tomatoes, chopped
1/2 cup raisins
1 1/2 cups couscous
1/8 teaspoon salt
1/2 teaspoon pepper
1/4 cup cucumber

PREPARATION
Roast the peppers under a broiler; remove and cool. On a nonstick baking sheet sprayed with Pam, place eggplant slices in a single layer and bake at 425°F, remove from oven and cool. In the meantime, boil a large pot of water, add potatoes, reduce heat and simmer. In a large skillet bring the broth and vinegar to a simmer; add shallots, ginger, onion, cumin, coriander, basil, cinnamon, and saffron. Simmer until the liquid almost evaporates. Stir in peppers and chickpeas and mix thoroughly. Add tomatoes, stirring until reduced to a thick sauce. Stir in the raisins, eggplant, and potatoes. Reduce heat to a simmer and cover. Cook for 10 minutes. Add two tablespoons of broth at a

time to prevent scorching. In the meantime prepare couscous. In a medium saucepan bring 1 3/4 cups of water to a boil. Place couscous in a large pot. Pour the boiling water over the couscous, cover and let stand for 20 minutes. Fluff with a fork; transfer to a serving platter. Make a deep well in the center and place skillet contents into it. Season with salt and pepper. Garnish with grated cucumber.

Prep time: 2 hours. Serves 4.

Notes:

Ratatouille

If you love eggplant, this is a wonderful way to prepare it. We enjoy it served over pasta. It freezes well and retains all of the rich flavor.

SHOPPING LIST
4 medium eggplants, sliced 1/4" thick
2 tablespoons extra virgin olive oil
4 onions, sliced
2 fennel bulbs, chopped
8 garlic cloves, crushed
2 each red, yellow, green bell peppers, roasted and sliced
12 medium ripe tomatoes, peeled, seeded, and chopped
6 parsley sprigs
2 thyme sprigs
2 bay leaves
1 rosemary sprig
2 firm zucchini, sliced 1/4" thick
1/8 teaspoon salt
1/4 teaspoon pepper

PREPARATION
On a nonstick baking sheet sprayed with Pam, place eggplant slices in a single layer and bake at 425° F, until browned on top. Turn, remove from oven, and cool. Heat oil in a large skillet; add onions, fennel, and garlic. Sauté, stirring often. Wrap spices in cheesecloth and secure with string. Stir in bell peppers, eggplant, tomatoes, and spice ball. Simmer gently for about 25 minutes, until the sauce thickens. Stir in zucchini and cook until tender. Remove spice ball, season with salt and pepper. May be served warm or cold.

Prep time: 1 1/4 hours. Serves 8.

Notes:

Gabi's Olive, Bean, and Potato Stew

SHOPPING LIST

6 medium new potatoes
1 tablespoon extra virgin oil
2 large onions, chopped
2 garlic cloves, crushed
1 tablespoon oregano
1 tablespoon fresh basil
2 tablespoons dry white wine (Chardonnay)
2 cups tomatoes, chopped
2 cups cooked chickpeas
2 cups cooked white beans
8 pitted black olives
4 green olives
1 tablespoon grated Romano cheese
1/8 teaspoon salt
1/4 teaspoon pepper, freshly-ground

PREPARATION

In a large stockpot gently simmer potatoes in water until just cooked through, about 12 minutes. Lift potatoes out of water and cool. Heat the oil in a large skillet; add onions, garlic, oregano, and basil. Sauté until onions are tender. Add wine, stir, and cook to reduce. Stir in tomatoes. Stir often until mixture starts to thicken. Add peas, beans, and olives. Dice potatoes and add to mixture. Cover and continue to cook, stirring occasionally until thick. Season with salt and pepper. Sprinkle the top with cheese and serve.

Prep time: 45 minutes. Serves 6.

Notes:

Snuffy's Porcine Mushroom and Lentil Stew

This is a treat for your friends who think you need meat to make a meal.

SHOPPING LIST

1 ounce dried porcine mushrooms
2 1/2 large onions
1 cup lentils
1 bay leaf
2 tablespoons extra virgin olive oil
4 garlic cloves, crushed
2 leeks, chopped
1/4 cup cilantro, chopped
2 teaspoons ground cumin
1/2 teaspoon coriander
1 teaspoon cinnamon
2 tablespoons balsamic vinegar
2 cups shiitake mushrooms
2 parsnips, peeled and sliced
1 tablespoon whole-wheat flour
1 pound firm tofu
1 teaspoon tobasco sauce

PREPARATION

Rehydrate porcine mushrooms by adding hot water to cover. This takes about 30 minutes. Chop one onion and set aside. Cut the remaining onions into quarters and put in a large saucepan. Add the lentils, bay leaf, and enough water to cover. Bring to a boil, cover, reduce heat, and simmer for 30 minutes. In the meantime heat oil in a 10-inch skillet; add chopped onion, leeks, garlic, and spices. Sauté until the vegetables are tender. Add vinegar and stir. Add fresh mushrooms and parsnips, and cook until tender. Drain porcine mushrooms reserving the liquid. Chop them and add to the skillet. Sprinkle the flour over the mixture and stir well. Drain lentils, discard bay leaf, and add lentils to mushroom mixture. Stir in the reserved mushroom liquid and continue to stir until mixture thickens. Add tofu and stir until well coated. Cover and simmer for 45 minutes. Garnish with cilantro.

Prep time: 1 3/4 Hours. Serves 6.

Notes:

144

Spaghetti with Variations

SHOPPING LIST
1 pound spaghetti (#9)
1 quart tomato sauce (Classico)
1 tablespoon basil
1 tablespoon oregano
1 tablespoon coriander
5 garlic cloves, crushed
1/4 teaspoon black pepper, crushed

PREPARATION
Bring 3 quarts of water to a boil. Add the pasta and cook until *al dente*, drain. Heat the Classico sauce over very low heat. Add the spices and garlic. Pour over the pasta and toss to thoroughly coat.

Variations
Prepare as above with the following ingredients.

SHOPPING LIST
1 pound spaghetti (#9)
1 quart tomato sauce (Classico)

Variation
1 cup chopped fresh tomatoes, chopped, or
1 cup cooked garbanzo beans,
1 cup cooked lentils, or
1 cup tofu, chopped (browned in Pam)
1 tablespoon basil
1 tablespoon oregano
1 tablespoon coriander
5 garlic cloves, crushed
1/4 teaspoon black pepper, crushed

More Variations

SHOPPING LIST
10 to 12 ripe tomatoes, or 2 15 1/2-ounce cans tomatoes, chopped
1 tablespoon olive oil
1/2 cup fresh basil
6 garlic cloves, crushed
2 cups cooked or 1 15 1/2-ounce can garbanzo beans,
    rinsed and drained
1 teaspoon oregano

PREPARATION

Blanche tomatoes, remove skins, and seeds. Put in a saucepan and add spices, garlic, and oil. Heat gently over low heat. Meanwhile, blend the garbanzo beans in a food processor until smooth. Add the beans to the sauce, stirring in gently over low heat. Pour over pasta and toss to coat.

Prep time: 45 minutes. Serves 4.

Notes:

Rose's Surefire Meatless Meatballs

When you taste these meatballs you won't believe they are made of tofu. But best of all, they taste good. The spices make the dish. Tofu is bland, and takes on any flavor.

SHOPPING LIST
1 pound silken tofu
1 cup whole-wheat breadcrumbs
1 tablespoon oregano
1 tablespoon basil
1 tablespoon coriander, ground
1/8 teaspoon salt
1/2 teaspoon black pepper
5 garlic cloves, crushed
1 teaspoon powdered garlic
1/2 cup Eggbeaters

PREPARATION
In a large bowl mash tofu and slowly add Eggbeaters and other ingredients. Mix very well. Mixture should be slightly dry. Form into one-inch balls and brown in a nonstick skillet with Pam or a small amount of olive oil. Alternatively, bake in a 400° F oven until brown. Add to the spaghetti sauce and serve over pasta.

Prep time: 20 minutes. Serves 6.

Notes:

Our Best Vegetarian Chili

We always soak our beans overnight. We change the water at least twice and cook the beans in fresh water. This helps eliminate any discomfort some people experience when eating beans, and keeps the sodium to a minimum. You can control the heat, by adding or subtracting the peppers!! Enjoy!

SHOPPING LIST

1/2 cup water or miso
1/2 cup onion, chopped
1/2 cup green bell pepper, chopped
1/2 cup zucchini, chunked
1/2 cup yellow straight-necked squash, chunked
1/2 cup corn, frozen
1 28-ounce can stewed tomatoes
1 tablespoon soy sauce
1/2 pound firm tofu, drained and chunked
1 cup black soy beans, cooked
1 cup pinto beans, cooked
1 cup white beans, cooked
1 cup green chilies, chopped (more if you're brave!)
1 tablespoon chili powder
1/8 teaspoon cayenne powder

PREPARATION

Put broth, onion, and green pepper in a large stockpot. Cook and stir about 5 minutes, until the onion is tender. Add the remaining ingredients, stir to mix well, and bring to a boil. Reduce heat and cook uncovered over medium-low heat for 30 minutes. Serve in soup bowls over whole grains. Excellent with a mixture of brown and wild rice.

Prep time: 1 hour. Serves 8.

Notes:

Kevan's Free Union Pie

This dish will remind you of meat and potatoes—without the meat. It is delicious and will satisfy even the hungriest of appetites. So dig in and add a glass of burgundy and a slice of crusty bread.

SHOPPING LIST
4 potatoes, peeled and diced
3/4 cup mung beans
2 leeks, diced
2 carrots, diced
1 cup frozen corn
2 tablespoons ginger, finely-grated
1/2 teaspoon dried dill
1 tablespoon apple juice
1 teaspoon miso

PREPARATION
Boil and then mash potatoes. In a separate pan cover the mung beans with water and boil for 15 to 20 minutes. Spray an ovenproof casserole dish with Olive Oil Pam and put in leeks, carrots, corn, dill, ginger, and apple juice. Mix well. Drain the beans, reserving the stock, and add the beans to the casserole. Dissolve the miso in some of the bean stock and add to the casserole. Cover and cook in the oven at 400° F for 45 minutes, stirring a few times. Add more bean stock if necessary. Remove from the oven and cover the casserole with a layer of the mashed potatoes to make the pie. Place under the broiler to brown.

Prep time: 20 minutes. Total time: 70 minutes. Serves 4.

Notes:

Main Courses

Garbanzo Bean Burgers

To cook burgers on the gas or charcoal grill, just add a sheet of aluminum foil or a barbecue grill screen, usually made of perforated metal, to keep them from coming apart in the process.

SHOPPING LIST
2 cups garbanzo beans, cooked
1 carrot, finely-chopped
1 celery stalk, finely-chopped
1/2 cup onion, finely-chopped
1 egg white
1/4 cup whole-wheat flour
1/8 teaspoon salt
1/4 teaspoon pepper

PREPARATION
In a food processor coarsely blend the garbanzo beans. Put in a bowl and add the remaining ingredients. Mix thoroughly. Form patties and fry in a nonstick skillet coated with Olive Oil Pam over medium heat. Brown on both sides. Remove and serve on whole-wheat buns or between toasted whole-wheat bread slices. Garnish with lettuce and tomato, if desired.

Prep time: 25 minutes. Serves 4 to 6.

Variation:
Add 1 ounce of silken tofu to the mixture.

Notes:

Lasagna

Lasagna is an Italian's version of a New York strip steak. We serve it for very special occasions. Now that we have discovered how to make this "sinful" dish without the fat, we enjoy it and pretend we are still sinning.

SHOPPING LIST

1 pound lasagna noodles, whole-wheat, or spinach
1 1/2 pints nonfat ricotta cheese or 12 ounces of soft tofu
1 pound nonfat mozzarella cheese
1/2 cup nonfat Parmesan
1 tablespoon dill
1/2 cup Eggbeaters
1 1/2 pints tomato sauce

PREPARATION

Cook noodles, using package directions. Drain. In a small bowl mix the ricotta cheese with the dill and Eggbeaters. In a large, rectangular baking pan, sprayed lightly with Olive Oil Pam, ladle sauce to cover the bottom. Layer noodles followed by sauce and mozzarella cheese. Add another layer of noodles and spoon and smoothe the ricotta cheese mixture over the top. Add more sauce and repeat the layers twice. Over the final layer of noodles add sauce and sprinkle the Parmesan cheese. Cover with aluminum foil and bake for 40 minutes in a 400° F oven. Remove the foil and bake for 10 minutes more. Let stand for 10 minutes and serve.

Prep time: 1/2 hour. Total time: 2 hours. Serves 6.

Notes:

Vegan Lasagna

As if taking out the fat is not enough, we now take out the animal. We hope you love this one. Experiment with your own variations.

SHOPPING LIST

3/4 cup water
1 tablespoon reduced-sodium soy sauce
1 onion, chopped
4 garlic cloves, crushed
1 28-ounce can crushed tomatoes
1 6-ounce can tomato paste
2 teaspoons basil
1 teaspoon oregano
1/2 teaspoon thyme
1 teaspoon fennel seeds
1/2 teaspoon black pepper
1 pound firm tofu, mashed
1/4 teaspoon salt
1/2 teaspoon nutmeg
1/2 teaspoon cinnamon
1/2 teaspoon black pepper
1 15-ounce can garbanzo beans, drained and processed smoothe
1/2 cup fresh dill, chopped
1 10-ounce frozen chopped spinach, thawed
1 8-ounce package Italian-style Vegan/Rella, grated
1-pound package lasagna noodles

PREPARATION

In a pot of boiling water cook the noodles *al dente*, about 5 minutes. Heat the water and soy sauce in a large skillet, add onion and garlic, and cook over medium-high heat until the onion is tender. Add the tomatoes, tomato paste, and spices. Simmer for 15 minutes. Preheat the oven to 350° F. Combine the mashed tofu, salt, nutmeg, cinnamon, and black pepper. Set aside.

Add the dill to the processed garbanzo beans and mix. To assemble the lasagna spread 1 cup of the sauce in a 9 x 12 inch pan. Cover the bottom with a layer of noodles. Next, layer the tofu mixture, spinach, Vegan/Rella, and the bean mixture.

Repeat layering twice. End with the noodles and a layer of sauce. Cover with foil and bake for 30 minutes. Let stand for 10 minutes before serving.

Prep time: 1 1/4 hours. Serves 10 to 12.

Variation

Substitute no-boil lasagna noodles or San Giorgio's Oven Ready Lasagne Pasta.

Notes:

Louise's Summer Casserole

Sara often takes this to a covered-dish supper. Prepare the night before and reheat in a microwave oven at the supper location.

SHOPPING LIST

1 eggplant, unpeeled, sliced 1/3" thick
1 large ripe tomato, thinly-sliced
3 large hard-boiled egg whites, sliced
1/2 cup shredded nonfat mozzarella
1 cup fresh breadcrumbs
1/2 cup grated Romano
3 garlic cloves, crushed
3 tablespoons fresh basil, minced
3 tablespoons fresh parsley, minced
1 teaspoon oregano
1/3 cup black olives
1 tablespoon extra virgin olive oil

PREPARATION

Heat oven to 425° F. Spread the eggplant slices in a single layer on a nonstick baking sheet and bake until tender. Spray an 8-inch baking dish with Olive Oil Pam. Remove the eggplant from the oven and transfer the slices to the baking dish, covering the bottom, overlapping if necessary. Layer the tomatoes next; then distribute the cheese and eggs on the top. In a food processor or blender, combine breadcrumbs, Romano cheese, garlic, basil, oregano, parsley, and olives. Sprinkle evenly over the baking dish of ingredients, and drizzle with olive oil. Cover with foil and bake for 15 minutes. Remove the foil and continue baking until the cheese is melted. About 10 minutes. Let stand before serving.

Serve hot or cold.

Prep time: 2 1/2 hours. Serves 4.

Notes:

Judi's Zucchini Parmesan Casserole

This is another Smith Mountain Lake Classic. The vacationers' delight. The first version of this recipe is very easy to prepare, leaving plenty of time to do other things in the kitchen before it is ready. The second version is more labor-intensive, but takes less time from start to serve.

SHOPPING LIST
3 tablespoons olive oil
1 cup onion, chopped
8 garlic cloves, crushed
3 cups zucchini, chunked
1 1/2 cups chopped plum tomatoes, with juice
1 1/2 cups cooked beans, mixture of red kidney, garbanzo, northern white
1/4 cup fresh basil
2 teaspoons fresh thyme
1/2 cup grated low-fat Parmesan or Romano cheese
salt and freshly-ground black pepper to taste

PREPARATION
Version 1:
Preheat the oven to 350° F. In a large bowl thoroughly mix all ingredients, except the cheese. Place the mixture in a casserole dish previously sprayed with Olive Oil Pam. Bake for 35 minutes. Remove from the oven and stir the cheese into the mixture. Return to the oven. Bake until the cheese browns. Remove from the oven and serve.

Prep time: 1 1/4 hours. Serves six.

We often mix version one and prepare for the freezer. It will keep for two months. We thaw the casserole for two hours before putting it in the oven. After 20 minutes stir the mixture and return to the oven. Proceed as directed.

Version 2:
Heat the oil in a nonstick skillet, add the zucchini and sauté until lightly browned. Remove the zucchini from the skillet and set aside. Preheat the broiler. Add the garlic and onions to the skillet and cook until translucent. Add the tomatoes, spices, beans, and zucchini. Bring to a simmer and continue to cook for 7 minutes. Mix in the cheese and place in a previously-sprayed baking dish.

Place under the broiler until the cheese is browned. Remove and serve.

Prep time: 45 minutes. Serves 6.

Notes:

Poultry and Seafood Dishes

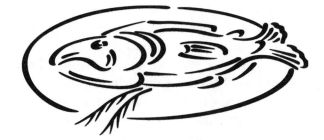

Maryland Crab Cakes

We first discovered this recipe on Ocracoke Island at the Back Porch. However, the islanders' variation has real eggs, real mayo, and lots of fat. Do we miss it?

SHOPPING LIST
8 ounces jumbo lump blue crabmeat
8 ounces back-fin blue crabmeat
5 to 8 slices day-old whole-wheat bread, crust removed
4 ounces Eggbeaters
1/2 cup nonfat mayonnaise
1/2 teaspoon Worcestershire sauce
1 teaspoon Dijon mustard
1/2 teaspoon lemon zest
1/8 teaspoon salt
1/2 teaspoon pepper
1/2 cup fresh parsley, minced
1/2 cup fresh chives, snipped

PREPARATION
Examine crabmeat and remove small pieces of shell. In a food processor, process the bread into breadcrumbs. In a large bowl, whisk mayonnaise into the Eggbeaters. Add the Worcestershire sauce, mustard, lemon zest, salt, and pepper. Place half of the breadcrumbs on top of the crabmeat in another large bowl. Pour half of the egg mixture on top of this and gently mix together. If you like your cakes dry, add more breadcrumbs. If you like them moist, add more egg. Add the parsley and chives and blend. Form into 6 to 8 balls. Pat them slightly flat with your hand. Use the remaining breadcrumbs to coat the cakes and place on a coated baking sheet. Refrigerate for one hour. Preheat the oven to 400° F. Bake the cakes for 10 minutes; then turn and bake until golden brown on both sides.

Prep time: 45 minutes. Serves 6.

Notes:

Mediterranean Flavor Fish Stew

We like to serve this to our friends who love fish. It is an interesting way to prepare cod fish. We are sure it will be one of your favorites.

SHOPPING LIST
2 tablespoons olive oil
2 large onions, diced
6 garlic cloves, crushed
1/2 teaspoon ground fennel seeds
1/8 teaspoon ground cloves
1/2 teaspoon cinnamon
1/2 teaspoon saffron threads, dissolved in boiling water
1 28-ounce can peeled whole tomatoes, drained and chopped
   (reserve liquid)
3 medium yams or sweet potatoes, peeled and chunked
1 small butternut squash, peeled, seeded, and chunked
1 teaspoon grated orange peel
1 1/2 pounds codfish steak, rinsed, dried, and chunked
1 tablespoon fresh lemon juice
1/2 teaspoon black pepper, freshly-ground
1/4 cup fresh parsley, minced for garnish

PREPARATION
In a large pot heat the oil, add onions, and garlic. Stir until they are coated. Cover the pot. Cook the onions and garlic over low heat until they are very soft, stirring occasionally. Add the fennel and cloves and cook for a minute. Then add the saffron, tomatoes, potatoes, squash, orange peel, and the tomato liquid. Cook partially covered over medium heat until the vegetables are soft—about 15 minutes. Add the fish and cook until flaky. Season with lemon juice and pepper, and then garnish with the parsley and serve.

Prep time: 1 1/4 hours. Serves 6.

Notes:

Shrimp Patel

Shrimp Patel will remind you of the days of outlandish eating. Do you remember the days when we could hardly get up from the table? Well, forget them—now you can eat until you are full and still have calories to spare for the next meal.

SHOPPING LIST

2 pounds medium shrimp, peeled and deveined
2 large vidalia onions, sliced
2" piece of fresh ginger, peeled
1/4 cup lemon juice
2 tablespoons olive oil
1 tablespoon whole cloves
1 tablespoon black peppercorns
1 tablespoon fennel seeds
1 tablespoon mustard seeds
1 tablespoon coriander seeds
1 tablespoon cumin seeds
1 cup plain nonfat yogurt
1 1/2 cups brown basmati rice
1/3 cup soy milk
1/2 teaspoon saffron threads
1/2 cup golden raisins
1/3 cup carrot, shredded
1/4 cup English walnuts

PREPARATION

Quarter one onion and put into a food processor with the garlic, ginger, and lemon juice; pulse 5 times. Pour the mixture into a bowl. Thinly slice one onion; heat oil in a heavy skillet and sauté onion and next 6 spices until onion is soft. Remove from the heat; stir in yogurt and ginger mixture; blend thoroughly. Cover and refrigerate.

Preheat the oven to 350°F. Bring 4 cups water to a boil. Add the rice and simmer for 10 minutes. Drain in a strainer. In a decorative baking dish add the shrimp, sauce mixture, and pour the rice on top and smoothe.

In a small pan bring the soy milk and saffron to a simmer. Remove from the heat and let stand for 2 minutes. Pour the liquid in streaks over the rice, sprinkle with the raisins, cover and bake for 35 minutes. Garnish with the shredded carrot and nuts.

Prep time: 1 1/4 Hours. Serves 6.

Notes:

K.W.'s Bayou Shrimp Stew

K.W. loves any meal you can add a touch of the bayou to, but this is one of his favorites.

SHOPPING LIST
2 tablespoons virgin olive oil
3/4 cup whole-wheat flour
1 pound medium shrimp in the shells
2 1/2 cups onions, thinly-sliced
2 cups celery, thinly-sliced
1 cup green bell pepper, diced
1 cup yellow or red bell pepper, diced
1 cup scallions, chopped
1 cup fresh cilantro, chopped
1 large carrot, diced
4 garlic cloves, crushed
1 teaspoon thyme
4 cups cooked brown rice

PREPARATION
Make a sauce by heating the oil in a heavy pan. Slowly stir the flour into the oil until it begins to brown. Reduce heat and continue to cook, stirring often, for about 20 minutes. Peel and devein the shrimp. Save the shells. In a saucepan boil 4 cups of water. Add shrimp shells and cook for 20 minutes. Remove the shells and discard, reserving the stock. Spray a stockpot with Olive Oil Pam; then sauté onions, green peppers, carrots, and celery until tender. Add the sauce and stir. Slowly stir in the reserved shrimp stock. Add the garlic, red or yellow pepper, and thyme. Simmer for 30 minutes. Stir occasionally. Add shrimp, scallions, and cilantro and simmer for 5 minutes longer. Serve over warm brown rice.

Prep time: 1 1/2 hours. Serves 5.

Notes:

Orange Roughy with Lemon/Orange Sauce

Orange roughy is wonderful when cooked this way. It adds a special touch for an elegant meal.

SHOPPING LIST

Sauce
2 tablespoons orange juice
3 tablespoons lemon juice
2 teaspoons lemon zest
1 teaspoon dry mustard
1 1/2 tablespoons extra virgin olive oil
Pinch white pepper

Main Dish
8 green beans, cut on the diagonal
2 carrots, cut into fine sticks
2 pounds orange roughy fillets
1/2 teaspoon white pepper
2 scallions, thinly-sliced
2 shallots, finely-chopped
Skin of one lemon, cut into thin strips

PREPARATION

Preheat oven to 400° F. Spray Olive Oil Pam on a large enough baking dish to hold the fish in a single layer. In a small bowl, whisk together all sauce ingredients until well blended. Set aside. Bring a pot of water to a boil and add green beans and carrots; cook for 2 minutes, remove with a slotted spoon, and plunge them into ice water. Set aside. Rinse fish, pat it dry, and place it in the oiled baking dish. Cover with a lid or foil wrap. Bake until the fish is flaky, about 12 minutes. Transfer the fish to a warm serving platter. Sprinkle with the cooked vegetables, scallions, shallots, and lemon strips. Spoon the sauce over the fish and serve.

Prep time: 45 minutes. Serves 4.

Notes:

Baked Chicken with Variations

For those of us who love chicken, these recipes are lifesavers. They have no fat added and are delicious. Enjoy!

SHOPPING LIST

4 chicken breasts, deboned and skinned
1/2 cup whole-wheat breadcrumbs
1 tablespoon powdered garlic
1 tablespoon oregano
1 tablespoon basil
1 tablespoon coriander
1/2 cup Eggbeaters

PREPARATION

Wash and dry the chicken and remove all fat. Preheat oven to 400° F. Mix breadcrumbs with spices in a shallow bowl. In another shallow bowl, whisk Eggbeaters. Coat chicken with Eggbeaters and then with the breadcrumbs. Put in a baking dish or pan, coated with Olive Oil Pam. Bake in a 400° F oven. Turn and brown on both sides, approximately 15 minutes each.

Prep time: 45 minutes. Serves 4 to 6.

Variation 1

SHOPPING LIST

4 chicken breasts, deboned and skinned
1/2 cup Grape Nuts, finely-crushed
1 tablespoon powdered garlic
1 tablespoon oregano
1 tablespoon basil
1 tablespoon coriander
1/2 cup Eggbeaters

PREPARATION

Wash and dry chicken and remove all fat. Preheat oven to 400° F. Mix the Grape Nuts with spices in a shallow bowl. In another shallow bowl whisk Eggbeaters. Coat chicken with Eggbeaters and then with Grape Nuts. Put in a baking dish or pan, coated with Olive Oil Pam. Bake in a 400°F oven. Turn and brown on both sides, approximately 15 minutes each.

Prep time: 45 minutes. Serves 4 to 6.

Variation 2

SHOPPING LIST

1 pound chicken tenders
1/2 cup corn flakes, finely-crushed
1 tablespoon powdered garlic
1 tablespoon oregano
1 tablespoon basil
1 tablespoon coriander
1/2 cup Eggbeaters

PREPARATION

Wash and dry the chicken and remove gristle, if any. Preheat oven to 400° F. Mix corn flakes with spices in a shallow bowl. In another shallow bowl whisk Eggbeaters. Coat chicken with Eggbeaters and then with corn flakes. Put in a baking dish or pan, coated with Olive Oil Pam. Bake in a 400° F oven. Turn and brown on both sides, approximately 15 minutes each.

Prep time: 45 minutes. Serves 4.

Notes:

Poultry & Seafood Dishes

Peachy Chicken

Peachy chicken is a tasty and sophisticated main course. Complemented by vegetables, a starch, and a salad, this is excellent company fare. Children love this dish, enticed by the fruit.

SHOPPING LIST

4 chicken breasts, deboned and skinned
Pam Olive Oil spray
1 teaspoon cinnamon
1/2 teaspoon nutmeg
1 15-ounce can peaches in light syrup
1 8-ounce can mandarin oranges
2 cups brown basmati rice, cooked

PREPARATION

Wash and dry chicken and remove all fat. In a skillet sprayed with Olive Oil Pam, brown chicken on both sides. Add peaches, cinnamon, and nutmeg; cook covered, over low heat, for 30 minutes. Add oranges and cook for 5 more minutes. Serve over brown rice.

Prep time: 1 1/4 hours. Serves 4.

Notes:

Poached Chicken

Poached chicken is a simple, but elegant dish. For those who like a light flavored meal, this is just the ticket.

SHOPPING LIST

4 chicken breasts, deboned and skinned
2 cups water
2 cups dry white wine
1 tablespoon thyme
1 small onion, quartered
1/2 teaspoon rosemary

PREPARATION

In a stockpot bring the water, wine, onion, and spices to a boil. Cook for 7 minutes uncovered. Add chicken breasts, cover pot, and simmer for 25 minutes.

Prep time: 35 minutes. Serves 4.

Notes:

Poultry & Seafood Dishes

Ginny's Salmon

Ginny's Salmon is a very simple and wonderful meal. Anytime you must make an elegant meal quickly, open your book to this recipe. You'll have rave reviews from your guests.

SHOPPING LIST
1 to 3 pounds whole fresh cleaned salmon (remove head and tail)
1/2 cup of fresh dill, minced
1/4 teaspoon salt
1/2 teaspoon black pepper
1 large lemon, very thinly sliced
1 teaspoon olive oil

PREPARATION
Preheat oven to 350° F. Wash and dry salmon; season with dill, salt, pepper, and olive oil. Place in a foil envelope and lay thin slices of lemon on both sides of the fish. Close and tightly seal the foil. Place in a baking dish or pan. Bake for one hour. Remove from the oven and let stand for 5 minutes. Lay salmon on a serving dish lined with parsley or dill. Serve with a nonfat yogurt sauce or freshly sliced lemons.

Prep time: 1 1/2 hours. Serves 4 to 10.

This method can be used with chicken or other fish.

Notes:

Steve's Grilled Salmon

This recipe mingles the wonderful flavors of fresh salmon with fresh herbs. Add vegetables to provide an eye appealing and wonderfully tasty center of attraction for an informal luncheon or dinner. Serving a whole salmon provides a glorious visual focal point on any table; but is easiest and, therefore, most appropriate to serve at a buffet meal. Since fresh salmon is now available all year long, consider this recipe for summer as well as winter occasions. It seems most appropriate at Thanksgiving Dinner as the Pilgrims probably consumed far more salmon in the early days than they consumed of the elusive wild turkey. Salmon is one of nature's best sources of omega-3 fatty acids, which can provide health benefits for all.

SHOPPING LIST
1 whole fresh salmon (optional: remove head)
Dry marinade:
    1 tablespoon salt (optional)
    1/4 cup brown sugar
    1 tablespoon white pepper

Cooking broth:
6 garlic cloves, peeled and crushed
1 ounce ginger, peeled and sliced into quarter-size pieces
6 green onions, cleaned and cut lengthwise
4 carrots, cleaned, peeled, and cut thin lengthwise
4 stalks celery, cleaned and cut lengthwise
Bouquet of fresh herbs, discussed below
1 large, Myers lemon, juiced
2 cups distilled water (tap water may contain minerals which
    discolor fish.)

PREPARATION:
Eight to 10 hours in advance, scale, wash, and pat dry salmon. Mix the dry marinade and wipe into the salmon cavity. Refrigerate the marinating salmon for 4 to 8 hours. Remove salmon from the refrigerator about one-half hour before cooking to bring it to room temperature. Dry off exterior of fish and wipe out cavity, removing any excess marinade. (Do not rinse the fish again as it will absorb some of the rinse water.)

Herb Bouquets:
4-5 large sprigs basil
5 small sprigs oregano
5 small sprigs thyme
8 large sprigs parsley
1 large sprig rosemary

Warm grill on high. When very hot, reduce the grill setting(s) to low. Form a large sheet of aluminum foil into a baking sheet sufficiently large to hold the fish, liquid, herbs, and vegetables. Pour one cup of the water with the lemon juice into the aluminum foil baking sheet. Add the fish to water, then add the sliced vegetables and the herbs. The herbs and vegetables should be spaced evenly around the fish. At this point, close the grill and wait. Replenish the cooking broth as it evaporates.

Cooking time for this dish is an art, dependent on the size of the fish and the heat of your grill. The objective is for the side of the fish facing the grill to be mostly cooked when the fish is carefully turned onto the other side. This is done when the skin on the grill-facing side could easily be removed from the fish. This should have taken approximately 45 minutes.

The second side is likewise done when the skin on the second side is easily loosened from the fish, or about 30 minutes later. When both sides have been cooked, carefully remove the skin from the upward facing side of the fish. Remove the fish from the "pan" gently using several wide spatulas and place it on a serving platter skinned-side down. Remove the remaining skin from the fish. Another way to remove the fish from the foil is to first remove the cooking broth, herbs, and vegetables from the foil and place the serving platter over the skinned-side of the fish. The platter, fish, and foil are then turned over and the skin from the second side is removed. When served, garnish the fish with fresh herbs and serve. The flesh will easily lift off salmon with a wide fish serving fork.

Although the grilled salmon can be frozen, it doesn't seem to taste as good when defrosted; so send any leftovers home with your guests. They will thank you for it. By the way, the residual broth is delicious for use as a soup or sauce base.

Prep time: 2 hours. Total time: 8 to 10 hours. Serves 6 to 8.

Notes:

Buck Mountain Squash Stew

This recipe was inspired by Stacy's love of squash and garbanzo beans. It is a favorite of ours.

SHOPPING LIST

2 tablespoons olive oil
4 cloves garlic, minced
2 medium onions, chopped
1 Jalapeno pepper, roasted, peeled, seeded, minced
1 Habnero pepper, roasted, peeled, seeded, minced
2 teaspoons fresh ginger, minced
1/2 teaspoon Hungarian paprika
1/2 teaspoon coriander
1/2 teaspoon ground cumin
1 butternut squash (1 1/2 to 2 pounds), peeled, seeded, cut into
    1-inch cubes
1 1/2 cups cooked or canned garbanzo beans, drained
1/2 cup golden raisins
3/4 cup apple juice
1 1/2 to 2 cups vegetable or chicken stock
3 cups spinach or chard, coarsely-chopped

PREPARATION

Heat oil in a 5-quart Dutch oven, add garlic and onion and sauté over very low heat, stirring frequently until golden and slightly caramelized. Add peppers and spices and sauté for 1 minute, or until spices are fragrant. Add squash, beans, raisins, apple juice, and 1 1/2 cups of the stock, stirring to combine. Bring to a boil, then cover pan and simmer over low heat until squash is almost tender but still firm. Stir occasionally during cooking. If liquid is absorbed, add more stock to keep vegetables moist. Add spinach (or chard) and more stock if needed. Cover and simmer until spinach or chard is tender.

Prep time: 1 1/4 hours. Serves 6.

Notes:

Sara's Meatless Meatloaf

Many people like meatloaf because it is such a homey meal. Now a vegetarian can enjoy a meatless meatloaf by using ground Boca. We have found it in vegetarian or natural food stores and also in large supermarkets.

SHOPPING LIST

1 12-ounce package ground Boca
1 1/2 cups cooked lentils
1 onion, chopped
3 celery stalks, chopped
2 carrots, chopped
2 garlic cloves, chopped
1 teaspoon basil
1 teaspoon oregano
2 tablespoons olive oil
3 egg whites
1 4-ounce package Eggbeaters
Salt and pepper to taste

PREPARATION

Sauté onion, garlic, celery, and carrot in olive oil until *al dente*. In a bowl combine ground boca, lentils, vegetables, and seasoning. Beat egg whites until slightly frothy. Add Eggbeaters to the Boca mix; then gently stir in the eggwhites. Lightly spray a loaf pan with Olive Oil Pam. Transfer mixture to pan and shape. Bake at 350° F for 30 minutes.

Prep time: 1 hour. Total time 1 1/2 hours. Serves 4.

Notes:

Chapter 13:

Side Dishes

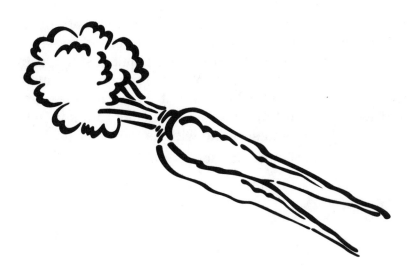

Oat Bran Risotto

Oat Bran Risotto is a savory blend of rice and mushrooms enhanced by the flavor of garlic, parsley, and onion. It is a wonderful accompaniment to any meal.

SHOPPING LIST
1 tablespoon olive oil
1 medium onion, finely chopped
3 garlic cloves, crushed
1/4 pound shiitake mushrooms, sliced
3 cups chicken stock
1 cup oat bran
1 cup long grain brown rice, cooked
Black pepper, freshly-ground
Parsley, chopped

PREPARATION:
Heat oil in large saucepan over medium-low heat. Add the onion and cook for one minute. Add the garlic and cook for four minutes. Push the mixture to the outer edges of the pan and raise the heat to medium. Add the mushrooms and cook, stirring often, until slightly browned. Stir in the chicken stock, scraping the sides and bottom of the pan. Whisk in the oat bran and cook, whisking constantly until thick, about 2 to 3 minutes. Stir the cooked rice into the bran mixture. Transfer to a serving dish, season with pepper, and sprinkle with parsley.

Prep time: 1 1/2 hours. If rice is pre-cooked, 45 minutes. Serves 4.

Notes:

Garlic Mashed with Wilted Greens

This dish is a splendid blend of greens and millet. The garlic and olive oil bring out the flavor of the escarole.

SHOPPING LIST
1 pound of tender escarole
2 large garlic bulbs, roasted
2 cups millet, cooked
2 tablespoons extra virgin olive oil
1/8 teaspoon salt
1/2 teaspoon black pepper

PREPARATION
Remove the base of the greens (trim 1/2"). Rinse and dry. Bring a large pot of water to a boil. Drop in greens and cook for 5 minutes. Drain and spread in a single layer in a baking pan to cool. When cool, squeeze to remove as much moisture as possible. In the meantime, put garlic on a cookie sheet and bake at 400° F for 30 minutes. Remove from the oven and cool. Squeeze the garlic bulbs into the millet. Mash with a fork and season to taste. Rinse a medium-size bowl with cold water. Shake out water, leaving the bottom damp. Pack the warm millet into the bottom and sides of the bowl, leaving the center hollow. Mix the greens with the oil and seasonings and put into the hollow.

Prep time: 45 minutes. Serves 6.

Notes:

Quinoa Timbales

We looked for timbale cups for at least two years before finding them in a gourmet shop in Charlottesville, Va. They have made preparing this recipe a truly gourmet-looking as well as gourmet-tasting dish.

SHOPPING LIST

1 cup quinoa
1 medium onion, minced
1 tablespoon olive oil
1 teaspoon ground cumin
1/2 teaspoon cinnamon
1/4 teaspoon turmeric
1/2 teaspoon nutmeg
1/8 teaspoon salt
1 2/3 cups vegetable stock
1/3 cup golden raisins
1/4 cup tomatoes, drained and chopped
3 tablespoons fresh parsley, chopped

PREPARATION

Cook the onion in heated oil over moderately-low heat until onion is tender. Add the spices and cook the mixture, stirring for one minute. Add broth, raisins, quinoa, and salt. Cover and simmer the mixture until the liquid is absorbed. Stir in parsley. Divide among 6 lightly-oiled timbale molds, packing it firmly. Invert timbales onto a platter, garnish with greens, and serve.

Prep time: 1/2 hour. Serves 6.

Notes:

Artichokes a la Micheline

These artichokes, named for our mother, are one of Rose's staple starters. If you visit four times, she is likely to serve artichokes at least twice.

SHOPPING LIST

4 to 8 large artichokes
1/2 cup whole-wheat breadcrumbs
1 tablespoon granulated or powdered garlic
1 tablespoon oregano
1 tablespoon basil
1 tablespoon coriander, ground
1 tablespoon olive oil
1/4 cup grated Romano cheese (optional)

PREPARATION

Wash and dry artichokes. Trim tops about 1/2 inch. Spread leaves and place in a large pot. Fill pot 1 1/2 inches with vegetable stock. Sprinkle the breadcrumbs, spices, and cheese over the tops making sure they settle among the leaves. Drizzle the oil over the tops, and cover. Cook for one hour over low heat or until the bases of the leaves are tender. Remove to a serving dish and serve. Can be eaten hot or cold.

Prep time: 1 1/2 hours. Serves 4 to 8.

Notes:

Side Dishes

Grilled Vegetables

One summer we made variations of grilled vegetables almost everyday. We experimented until our hearts were content and our stomachs were full. Now we make this dish for our special guests.

SHOPPING LIST

1 medium eggplant
2 medium onions
1 large bell pepper
4 medium potatoes
2 leek stalks
2 fennel stalks
2 carrots
2 large shiitake mushrooms
3 tablespoons extra virgin olive oil
1/8 teaspoon salt
1/2 teaspoon black pepper
5 garlic cloves, crushed
1/4 cup fresh dill
1/4 cup fresh basil

PREPARATION

Clean the vegetables and slice in strips. Cook in microwave oven in a covered casserole dish for 5 minutes with 1/4 C water. Meanwhile blend the oil with the garlic, basil, dill, salt, and pepper. Marinate the vegetables in the blended oil. Let stand for 30 minutes. Drain and grill the vegetables until tender and brown on both sides. If a grill is not available, broil in the oven. When done, toss with the remainder of the blended oil and garnish with more fresh dill and/or basil.

Prep time: 30 minutes. Total time: 1 1/4 hours. Serves 4.

Notes:

Greens

Greens can be any one or a mixture of the following: dandelion, rapini, spinach, escarole, turnip greens, kale, or mustard. These greens can be served alone as a side dish or can be mixed with pasta, grains, or beans. They are a delicious and healthy dish.

SHOPPING LIST

2 pounds of greens
1 1/2 cups vegetable or chicken broth
6 garlic cloves, crushed and marinated in extra virgin olive oil
1/2 teaspoon basil, or oregano, or thyme, or rosemary, or lemon
  basil (optional)
1/8 teaspoon salt
1/2 teaspoon black pepper

PREPARATION

Trim and wash the greens in cold water. Tear into pieces and steam in boiling broth. Meanwhile, crush the garlic into the olive oil and let stand. When the greens are tender, remove from heat, and add oil, garlic, and spices.

Prep time: 20 minutes. Serves 6 to 8.

Notes:

Rapini Meanni

Rapini is a slightly bitter, but delicious, green. It adds spice to any meal.

SHOPPING LIST

1 pound rapini
1/2 cup shallots, thinly-sliced
1/2 teaspoon garam masala
1/2 teaspoon black pepper
1/2 teaspoon hot Hungarian paprika
2 cups low-sodium chicken broth

PREPARATION:

Heat the chicken broth, add the shallots and spices. Wash, chop the rapini, and add to the chicken broth. Cook until *al dente*. Remove from heat and serve in small bowls. If desired, sprinkle with Romano cheese.

Prep time: 15 minutes. Serves 4.

Notes:

Oven-Baked Potatoes

Oven-Baked Potatoes have become one of our favorite ways to serve potatoes. They are tasty and easy to make. Neither our families nor our guests ever leave one for tomorrow.

SHOPPING LIST
6 medium baking or sweet potatoes, scrubbed
Salt and pepper
Parsley

PREPARATION
Prick the potatoes with a fork. Place potatoes on oven rack in a 450° F oven. Bake until done, approximately 45 minutes. White potatoes can be served plain, or with nonfat sour cream, or yogurt, or a drizzle of olive oil. Sweet potatoes can be served plain or with fruit compote. Season to taste with salt, pepper, and parsley.

Prep time: 5 minutes. Total time: 50 minutes. Serves 6.

Notes:

Side Dishes

Oven-Browned Potatoes

SHOPPING LIST
6 medium baking potatoes, scrubbed
1/2 teaspoon each parsley, oregano, basil, and garlic

PREPARATION
Peel the potatoes, if you wish. Quarter and place in a baking dish that has been very lightly coated with Olive Oil Pam. Season with the spices and bake in a 450° F oven. Bake until done, approximately 35 minutes.

Prep time: 5 minutes. Total time: 40 minutes. Serves 6.

Notes:

Baked Onions

Baked Onions make a great substitute for baked potatoes. They just aren't starchy. This is our answer to the awesome onion blossom!!! This is so tasty that you will be able to indulge without taking in your weekly allowance of fat.

SHOPPING LIST
6 medium onions
1/2 teaspoon each parsley, oregano, basil, and garlic
1/2 cup breadcrumbs

PREPARATION
Peel onions and place in a baking dish that has been very lightly coated with Olive Oil Pam. Sprinkle onions with breadcrumbs, spices, salt, and pepper. Bake in an oven at 400° F. until soft, approximately 35 minutes.

Prep time: 5 minutes. Total time: 40 minutes. Serves 6.

Notes:

Side Dishes

Wease's Baked Beans

When we take these beans to a covered-dish supper, we never have a bean left.

SHOPPING LIST
1 32-ounce can butter beans
1 large onion, chopped
1/4 cup sugar
1 12-ounce bottle ketchup
Dash liquid smoke

PREPARATION
Mix sugar and onions in a glass casserole. Add beans, ketchup, and a dash of liquid smoke. Cover and bake at 350° F for 45 minutes.

Prep time: 1 hour. Serves 4 to 6.

Notes:

Roasted Tomato Casserole

We love to prepare this and serve it to the family or to guests. It is easy and delicious.

SHOPPING LIST

Dressing
4 garlic cloves, minced
2 tablespoons balsamic vinegar
2 teaspoons Dijon mustard
1/4 teaspoon salt
1/4 teaspoon pepper, freshly-ground
1/4 cup olive oil

Casserole
3 medium onions, sliced in thin rings
2 1/2 pounds (about 8 to 10) large tomatoes, thickly-sliced
3/4 cup fresh basil, chopped
2 1/2 tablespoons fresh oregano, chopped
1/2 cup fresh parsley, chopped
3 tablespoons breadcrumbs
3 tablespoons Romano cheese, freshly-grated

PREPARATION

Preheat oven to 375° F. Combine all dressing ingredients in a bottle, and shake to mix. Arrange half of the onions in a baking dish and sprinkle with 1 tablespoon of the dressing. Place half of the tomatoes over the onions and add another tablespoon of dressing. Combine herbs and sprinkle tomatoes with half of them. Repeat with another layer of onions, dressing, tomatoes, and herbs. Drizzle with remaining dressing. Combine breadcrumbs and cheese and sprinkle over tomatoes. Bake 1 hour. If tomatoes are too juicy, pour off excess liquid before serving.

Prep time: 1 1/2 hours. Serves 6.

Notes:

Side Dishes

Breakfasts

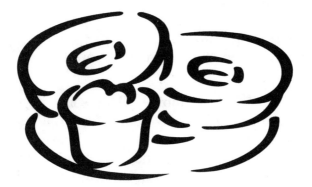

Oatmeal

This is a tradition with us almost every morning. We like it plain but you can really dress it up with dried or fresh fruits.

SHOPPING LIST

1 cup rolled oats
1 cup apple juice
1 cup water
1 tablespoon dried cranberries, or ginger marmalade,or raisins, or 1/2 cup fresh strawberries, or raspberries, or blueberries or 1 teaspoon ginger, freshly-grated
1 tablespoon honey or brown sugar

PREPARATION

Combine the oats, the liquids, and your choice of sweeteners and fruits in a large Pyrex bowl. Cook in microwave on highest power for three minutes, stir well, and cook for 4 to 5 minutes more on power level three. Stir and serve.

Prep time: 10 minutes. Serves 2 to 4.

Notes:

Sgarlat's Frittata

Frittatas are like omelets, but are easier to prepare. They do not require the precise timing or deftness of hand, and you only need one pan. You can make the filling and the frittata in the same skillet. You will really wow your guests who will think you were slaving in the kitchen.

SHOPPING LIST

1 4-ounce carton Eggbeaters
2 egg whites

Filling

1/2 cup nonfat grated or crumbled cheese (your choice)
1 cup vegetables (onions, mushrooms, spinach, red or green peppers, tomatoes), chopped
2 tablespoons fresh or dried herbs
1/2 cup leftover pasta

PREPARATION

Place a rack in the upper third of the oven and preheat the oven to 350° F. Lightly beat the egg whites into the Eggbeaters. Spray an ovenproof skillet lightly with Olive Oil Pam. Heat over medium-high heat on the stove. Put the filling of your choice into the pan; then pour the eggs over the filling. Stir lightly until the eggs start to set. Reduce the heat to medium low. Once the bottom is firm and about one-half inch thick, use a spatula to lift the edge of the frittata. Tilt the pan toward you so the uncooked egg runs underneath. Lower the edge and swirl the egg to distribute the egg. Continue cooking until the top is no longer runny. Put the skillet into the oven until the top is dry to the touch. Be careful not to overcook, because the eggs will be tough. Loosen the edges underneath the frittata and slide on to a serving plate. Season with salt and pepper. Serve hot, at room temperature, or chilled.

Prep time: 30 minutes. Serves 4.

Notes:

Rosie's French Toast

When you eat this French toast, we guarantee you will not miss the butter or the whole eggs. Add a touch of cinnamon for a different flavor, or add fruit to dress it up for company.

SHOPPING LIST

2 to 4 ounces Eggbeaters
1 tablespoon skim milk
8 slices whole-wheat bread
1 tablespoon maple syrup or honey

PREPARATION

Put the Eggbeaters into a shallow bowl, add the skim milk, and mix. Dip the bread into the egg mixture and coat on both sides. Brown on both sides in a nonstick skillet coated with Olive Oil Pam. Put on a serving plate and drizzle with warm syrup or honey.

Prep time: 15 minutes. Serves 4.

Notes:

Snuffy's Blueberry Pancakes

Snuffy is famous among our friends for this breakfast dish. In fact, we have eaten them for supper on more than one occasion.

SHOPPING LIST

Blueberry sauce
2 cups blueberries
1 cup white grape juice or apple juice
2 tablespoons cornstarch or arrowroot

Pancakes
1 1/2 cups whole-wheat flour
1 tablespoon sugar
11/2 teaspoons baking powder
3/4 teaspoon baking soda
2 large egg whites or 2 ounces Eggbeaters
1 1/2 cups nonfat buttermilk or plain nonfat yogurt
1 teaspoon vanilla extract
1 cup blueberries

PREPARATION

Sauce: In a saucepan heat the berries and the juice over low heat. Cook until the berries are soft; then add the cornstarch, which has been premixed with a tablespoon of water. Stir the berry mixture until thickened.

Pancakes: In a large bowl, mix the flour, sugar, baking soda, and powder. In a separate bowl, mix together egg whites or Eggbeaters, buttermilk or yogurt, and vanilla. Whisk wet ingredients into the dry ingredients until smooth. Stir in the blueberries. Coat a nonstick griddle or skillet with Olive Oil Pam and heat over medium-high. Drop batter, 1/4 cup at a time. Cook until bubbles form on the surface, flip, and cook the other side. Serve with blueberry sauce.

Prep time: 30 minutes. Serves 4.
Notes:

Diane's High Rise Waffles

High rise waffles are a wonderful treat to serve guests on a cold frosty morning. Serve them by the fireplace with hot chocolate or expresso.

SHOPPING LIST

1 cup unbleached all-purpose flour
1/8 teaspoon salt
1 teaspoon baking soda

2 ounces Eggbeaters

2 egg whites
1/4 cup nonfat buttermilk

PREPARATION

Spray the waffle iron with Olive Oil Pam and plug in to heat. Sift the flour, salt, and baking soda together in a large mixing bowl. In a separate bowl, lightly beat together Eggbeaters and buttermilk. Stir into the dry ingredients. Whip the egg whites until soft peaks form. Thoroughly fold the whites into the batter. Pour batter into the center of the waffle iron and cook until the indicator light goes out. Serve with the topping of your choice.

Prep time: 35 minutes. Serves 4.

Notes:

Rose's Omelet Delight

Though this dish is listed under breakfast foods, when we are in a hurry after a tiring day, we often serve it for dinner. A salad, crusty bread, and a glass of wine turn this into a splendid meal.

SHOPPING LIST
4-ounce carton Eggbeaters
1/2 cup mixture of onions, tomatoes, peppers finely-chopped
1/4 cup nonfat cheddar cheese
Salt and pepper, freshly-ground

PREPARATION
Precook the vegetables in the microwave oven for 1 minute. Spray a skillet with olive oil Pam and heat over medium heat. Slowly pour the egg into the skillet and reduce to low heat. When bottom forms, lift edge and let liquid seep underneath. Add in order: vegetables, cheese, salt, and pepper. Cover for 1 1/2 minutes. When the surface is dry, fold omelet and slide onto a serving dish.

Prep time: 12 minutes. Serves 2.

Notes:

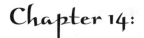

Chapter 14

Desserts

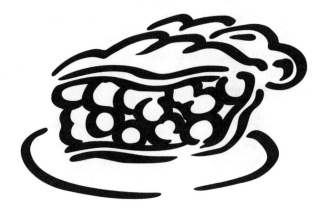

Wease's Stuffed Baked Apples

Come October, there is nothing like the smell of baked apples in our kitchen. This is a very healthy dessert. And what a treat!

SHOPPING LIST
4 medium baking apples
1/4 cup raisins
1/4 cup dried cranberries
2 tablespoons honey
1 tablespoon brown sugar
1 cup apple juice
1 teaspoon ground cinnamon
4 ounces nonfat vanilla yogurt

PREPARATION
Wash and partially core the apples. In a small bowl combine the fruits, brown sugar, honey, and 2 tablespoons of apple juice. Stuff the apple cavities with the fruit mixture. Pour the remaining apple juice into a baking dish and place the apples in it. Cover and bake for 40 minutes in a preheated 350° F oven. Remove from the oven and put a dab of yogurt on top of each apple and sprinkle with cinnamon.

Prep time: 1 hour. Serves 4.

Notes:

Rosie's Mixed Fruit

A dessert can't be simpler, and still taste as if we spent hours in preparation.

SHOPPING LIST

1 cup fresh or frozen raspberries
1 cup fresh or frozen strawberries
1 cup fresh or frozen blueberries
1 cup fresh pineapple
1 tablespoon sugar

Variations

1 tablespoon brandy
1 tablespoon cinnamon
1 tablespoon cointreau

PREPARATION

If using frozen berries, partially thaw and sprinkle with sugar and serve. If using fresh berries, clean, wash, and thoroughly drain. Add the sugar, mix, and let stand for one hour. Serve.

Prep time: 10 to 15 minutes. Total time: 1 1/4 hours. Serves 8.

Notes:

Rosie's Mixed Fruit over Angel Food Cake

For a more festive occasion.

SHOPPING LIST
1 cup fresh or frozen raspberries
1 cup fresh or frozen strawberries
1 cup fresh or frozen blueberries
1 cup fresh pineapple
1 tablespoon sugar

Variations
1 tablespoon brandy
1 tablespoon cinnamon
1 tablespoon cointreau
1 angel food cake

PREPARATION
If using frozen berries, partially thaw and sprinkle with sugar and spread over sliced angel food cake. If using fresh berries, clean, wash, and thoroughly drain. Add the sugar, mix, and let stand for one hour. Serve over sliced angel food cake.

Prep time: 10 to 15 minutes. Total time: 1 1/4 hours. Serves 8.

Notes:

Peach Crisp

Here is a dessert with no fat! And it tastes delicious. And the good news is that it is not a lot of work and does not take hours to prepare.

SHOPPING LIST

8 cups peaches, sliced
3 tablespoons tapioca
1 cup pineapple juice
2 tablespoons honey
1 teaspoon cinnamon

Crisp topping
1 1/3 cups rolled oats
1/2 cup whole-wheat flour
1/4 cup oat flour (to make, see Helpful Hints)
2 tablespoons honey
1/4 cup orange juice
1 teaspoon vanilla extract

PREPARATION

Preheat the oven to 375° F. Soften tapioca in pineapple juice in a small bowl for 5 minutes. Mix the tapioca into the remaining ingredients. Bake for 20 minutes. In the meantime make the topping. Combine the dry ingredients and the wet ingredients separately. Pour the liquid ingredients over the dry and toss to mix. Stir the peach mixture and crumble the topping over them. Bake for another 20 minutes.

Prep time: 1 1/4 Hours. Serves 6.

Any other kind of fruit may be substituted for the peaches.
Notes:

Carrot Cake

Now you can see that you do not need lots of fat and a lot of sugar to make a wonderful dessert.

SHOPPING LIST
1/2 cup carrots, grated
1/2 cup dates, chopped
1/2 cup raisins
1/2 cup dried cranberries
1 1/3 cups water
1/4 cup unsweetened applesauce
1 teaspoon cinnamon
1 teaspoon ground cloves
1 teaspoon nutmeg
1 teaspoon baking powder
1 teaspoon baking soda
2 cups whole-wheat flour

PREPARATION
Preheat the oven to 350° F. In a saucepan bring the carrots, dried fruits, water, applesauce, and spices to a boil. Reduce heat and simmer for 5 minutes. Cool. Mix dry ingredients together. Then combine wet and dry ingredients and stir until well blended. Spoon the batter into an 8" x 8" nonstick cake pan and bake for 45 minutes.

Prep time: 1 hour. Serves 4 to 8.

Notes:

Cheesecake a la Tofu

If you are a cheesecake fan, you will like this very much.

SHOPPING LIST

Crust

2 cups Grape Nuts cereal

1/3 cup frozen apple juice concentrate, thawed

Filling

2 pounds silken tofu

3/4 cup honey

1 teaspoon vanilla extract

1/2 teaspoon cinnamon

1/2 teaspoon nutmeg

Variation

1 ounce bakers' chocolate, melted

Topping

1 cup fresh or frozen berries or 1 fresh peach, thinly-sliced or
2 kiwi, sliced

PREPARATION

Blend the Grape Nuts to crush, place in a medium bowl, add the apple juice, and mix well. Press into a 9-inch pie plate and set aside. Mix the tofu and honey, add the vanilla, cinnamon, and nutmeg, and beat until fluffy with an electric mixer. Spoon into the pie shell and smoothe. Cover loosely with plastic wrap and refrigerate for 1 to 3 hours. Remove and cover the top with berries or fresh fruit slices. Serve.

Prep time: 45 minutes plus the time to chill. Serves 8 to 10.

Notes:

Rice Pudding

We have not met many people who do not like rice pudding. Pudding made with brown rice and low fat soy milk is a good choice.

SHOPPING LIST

4 cups brown rice, cooked
1 1/2 cups low-fat soy milk
1/2 cup golden raisins
2 tablespoons honey
1 teaspoon cinnamon
1 teaspoon vanilla extract

PREPARATION

Preheat oven to 325° F. Combine all ingredients in a bowl; then pour into a casserole. Bake for 45 minutes. Sprinkle the top with cinnamon. May be served hot or cold.

Prep time: 5 minutes. Total time: 55 minutes. Serves 4.

Notes:

Sara's Extra-Spicy Ginger Snaps

These are the spiciest ginger snaps we have ever baked, pleasing even our snappiest family and friends.

SHOPPING LIST

2 1/2 cups flour
2 teaspoons baking soda
3 teaspoons ground ginger
1 teaspoon ground cinnamon
1 1/2 teaspoons dry mustard
1 teaspoon white pepper
1 teaspoon ground cardamom
2 teaspoons ground cloves
1/4 teaspoon salt
3/4 cup apple butter
1 cup dark brown sugar, packed
2 ounces Eggbeaters
1/4 cup molasses
3 tablespoons granulated sugar

PREPARATION

Preheat oven to 350° F. Mix all dry ingredients, except sugars. On high speed mix apple butter and brown sugar until well blended. Add molasses and egg, then mix.

Reduce to medium speed and continue to mix for one minute. Add the flour mixture, beat on low, and then medium speed until well mixed. Divide dough in half, shape each half into a ball, wrap with plastic, and pat flat into a cake; then refrigerate for 1 to 2 hours or freeze for 20 minutes. Shape dough into 1-inch balls, roll in granulated sugar, and set at least 2 inches apart on a nonstick cookie sheet. Bake until dark brown on the bottom, about 5 minutes; then switch pan position and bake for 5 minutes more. Remove from oven, cool on sheet 5 minutes; then transfer to a rack and continue to cool. Store in an airtight container or eat them now.

Prep time: 30 minutes to prepare and bake, plus the time to cool the mixture. Serves 36 cookies.

Notes:

Desserts

Berryhill Green Tomato and Apple Pie

This is the solution to your "what to do with green tomatoes" problem. What a wonderful pie; it is not overly sweet. We gave a pie to a young man one day last fall and he told us he ate half of it before he got home! Make sure you have a true deep-dish pie plate to bake this pie.

SHOPPING LIST

Pastry for double-crust deep-dish 9-inch pie
2 1/2 tablespoons orange marmalade
1/2 cup dark brown sugar, firmly-packed
1/4 cup sugar
1/4 cup quick-cooking tapioca
1/2 cup raisins
1 teaspoon ground cinnamon
1/2 teaspoon ground ginger or 1 teaspoon of fresh ginger
1/4 teaspoon salt
6 medium green tomatoes, thinly-sliced
4 large Granny Smith apples, cored, peeled, and thinly-sliced
2 tablespoons applesauce

PREPARATION

Preheat oven to 425° F. Divide pastry in half; roll out one half; put in pie pan, leaving a 1-inch overhang. Spread marmalade evenly over bottom of pastry. In a small bowl, mix sugars, tapioca, raisins, cinnamon, ginger, and salt until well combined. Layer tomatoes, sugar mixture, and applesauce mixed with the apples until all ingredients are used. Roll out the remaining pastry and lay it over the filling. Crimp edges together to seal and make several small slits on top. Put pie pan on cookie sheet to catch drips. If desired, brush with milk and sprinkle with sugar before baking. Bake in preheated oven for 15 minutes at 425° F. Reduce heat to 325° F and bake 35 to 40 minutes longer.

Prep time: 1 1/2 hours. Serves 6 to 8.

Notes:

Terman's Soy Chocolate

The next two recipes, Terman's and Carson's, were sent to us by two subscribers to our newsletters. They taste just great, are easy to prepare, and will satisfy your sweet tooth.

SHOPPING LIST
4 squares of unsweetened chocolate
2 teaspoons vanilla
2 teaspoons lecithin
2 packages soybean instant drink
1 tablespoon brown sugar

PREPARATION
Melt chocolate in a double boiler; then mix in the remaining ingredients. Spread the mixture on waxed paper. Divide into squares with a knife. Refrigerate one hour or more.

Prep time: 20 minutes. Total time: 1 1/2 hours. Serves 4.

Notes:

Desserts

Carson's Strawberry Tofu Confection

SHOPPING LIST
1 pound tofu
6 ounces frozen strawberries
1 teaspoon sugar
2 ounces water

PREPARATION
In a blender, mix tofu and strawberries. Add sugar and water. Blend until smooth. Pour into four custard cups and refrigerate for at least an hour.

Prep time: 15 minutes. Total time 1 1/4 hours. Serves 4.

Notes:

Appendix 1

Herbs, Spices & Flavorings	Flavor	Fresh/Dried	Examples
Allspice	sweet aromatic	dried	baked fruit
Anise	licorice	fresh/dried	cookies
Basil	sweet	fresh/dried	tomatoes/pesto
Bay leaf		dried	soups/flour
Brown sugar	sweet/rich	dried	baked apples/ sweet potatoes/
Caraway	rye like	seeds	breads/soups
Cardamon	aromatic	dried powder	squash soup/stew
Cayenne	peppery/hot	dried	humus/chili/soups
Celery seed		seeds	soups/stews
Chili	peppery/hot	dried/powder	stews/chili
Chives	onion-like	fresh/dried	salads/sauces/dips
Cinnamon	pungent/aromatic	dried/stick/ground	drinks/cookies/ oatmeal/squash/soup
Cloves	pungent/aromatic	dried/whole/ ground	baked apples/ cookies/yams
Coriander/ cilantro	combination lemon peel and sage	dried/fresh/ ground/whole seeds	sauces/soups/ humus
Cumin	similar to caraway	dried/ground/ whole	chili/humus/ vegetables
Curry	pungent	dried	soups/rice/ vegetables
Dill	pungent	fresh/dried/seeds	cumbers/breads/ sauces
Fennel	anise/licorice	fresh/dried/seeds	salads/vegetables/ potatoes/tomatoes
Fenugreek	aromatic/pungent	dried/ground	salads/soups
Garlic	aromatic/pungent/ strong	fresh/ground	main dishes/ salads/ soups/vegetables
Ginger	pungent/spicy	fresh/ground	vegetables/salads/ soups/cookies
Lemon	fruity/bitter	fresh/concentrate	vegetables/main dishes/salads/ cookies
Marjoram	aromatic/sweet	dried leaves/ground	main dishes/ vegetables

Herbs, Spices & Flavorings	Flavor	Fresh/Dried	Examples
Mustard	hot/pungent/spicy	dried/whole seed	salads/main dishes
Nutmeg	fragrant/sweet/spicy	dried/whole/ground	fruit/cookies/squash/eggnog/sweet potatoes
Oregano	strong/aromatic/pleasantly bitter	fresh/dried	sauces/salads/main dishes
Paprika	sweet to hot/spicy red color	dried	chili/salads/vegetables
Parsley	mildly peppery	fresh/dried	salads/garnish/vegetables
Pepper (white/black)	hot/spicy	dried/ground/whole	salads/main dishes/soups/cookies
Poppy seed	pungent	seeds/ground	breads/vegetables/salads
Rosemary		fresh/dried	salads/main dishes
Saffron	bitter/pleasantly/yellow color	dried/ground/strings	vegetables/main dishes/curries
Sage	astringent/bitter/aromatic	fresh/dried/ground/rubbed	vegetables/main dishes/soups
Salt	salty	dried	salads/main dishes/vegetables/soups
Savory	pungent	fresh/dried	salads/soups/dressings/main dishes
Soy sauce	pungent/rich	liquid	soups/salads/main dishes
Tabasco	hot/peppery/spicy	liquid	soups/salads/main dishes
Tamari	pungent/rich	liquid	soups/salads/main dishes
Tarragon	piquant	fresh/dried leaves/ground	salads/main dishes
Thyme	aromatic/pungent	fresh/dried leaves/ground	salads/main dishes
Tumeric	bitter/aromatic	dried/ground	main dishes
Worchestershire sauce	spicy/peppery	liquid	main dishes

Appendix 2

BREADS

SOUPS

Main Courses

POULTRY AND FISH DISHES

SIDE DISHES

BREAKFASTS

DESSERTS

Appendix 3

Prostate Forum Newsletter

- Does prostate cancer affect you or someone you love?
- Are you bewildered by conflicting information about this disease?
- Do you find it difficult to get clear and accurate answers to your questions?

The *Prostate Forum*, written by Charles E. *Snuffy* Myers, Jr. MD is a monthly newsletter designed to answer your questions about prostate cancer. We have been publishing since June, 1996. Our subscribers think the *Prostate Forum* is the most informative newsletter written for patients and families. Every month we discuss important information that may affect your disease, quality of life, and survival.

The subscription fee is $36.00* a year.
Call 1 800-305-2432, FAX 804-974-9597 or send to:

Prostate Forum
Rivanna Health Publications, Inc.
P.O. Box 6696
Charlottesville, VA 22906-6696

Name: _____
          First   MI   Last

Address: _____

_____

City: _____

State: _____ Zip Code: _____

Phone: _____

Fax: _____

E-mail: _____

Delivery method: Please check one**
❑ E-mail   ❑ U.S. Mail

❑ Check enclosed: Payable to Rivanna Health Publications, Inc.
❑ Visa   ❑ MC

Account #: _____ Exp:_____

Signature: _____

*Funds must be in U.S. Add $10.00 for postage to CANADA and MEXICO. Add $36.00 for all other non-U.S. locations.
**If e-mail delivery is chosen, pay only the $36.00 subscription fee.